Praise for *Dreams of Awakening*:

'I have been involved in the Toltec culture of dreaming for many years and Charlie´s book is one of the best I have ever read about dreams. We are entering a new period of time in which the ancient lineages of dreamers were predicted to be rediscovered, and Charlie Morley is giving a treasure for these times, a modern view on the ancient Tibetan practices of dreaming.'
Sergio Magaña Ocelocoyotl, author of *2012–2021: The Dawn of the Sixth Sun*

'I have run joint retreats with Charlie and I consider him to be the most experienced and authentic practitioner of lucid dreaming teaching in Europe. He has been training since his teens and this book offers a training programme based on this unique practical experience.'
Rob Nairn, author of *Living, Dreaming, Dying*

'Joyfully exploring consciousness, lucid dreaming and Buddhism, Charlie Morley gently stretches the reader's mind to accept dream yoga's premise of real awakening. I recommend this for everyone on the lucid dreaming path..'
Robert Waggoner, author of *Lucid Dreaming: Gateway to the Inner Self*

'Charlie is proof of evolution. He's the next generation – sharp of mind and sweet of heart. He's like a DJ mixing old and new to create a practice that's relevant, useful and most importantly, one that works. I wholeheartedly recommend his book. He's the real thing.'
Ya'Acov Darling Khan, co-author of *Movement Medicine: How to Awaken, Dance and Live Your Dreams*

'This exciting book by a brilliant young teacher will enthral all those fascinated by the possibility of both lucid dreaming and lucid living.'
Tim Freke, author of *Lucid Living* and *The Mystery Experience*

To David,

Keep bending space-time!

DREAMS OF
AWAKENING

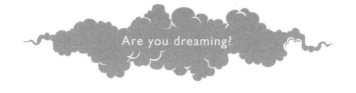

Are you dreaming?

With love & admiration,

Charlie
x x

DREAMS OF
AWAKENING

LUCID DREAMING AND MINDFULNESS OF DREAM & SLEEP

Are you dreaming?

CHARLIE MORLEY

HAY HOUSE

Carlsbad, California • New York City • London • Sydney
Johannesburg • Vancouver • Hong Kong • New Delhi

First published and distributed in the United Kingdom by:
Hay House UK Ltd, Astley House, 33 Notting Hill Gate, London W11 3JQ
Tel: +44 (0)20 3675 2450; Fax: +44 (0)20 3675 2451
www.hayhouse.co.uk

Published and distributed in the United States of America by:
Hay House Inc., PO Box 5100, Carlsbad, CA 92018-5100
Tel: (1) 760 431 7695 or (800) 654 5126
Fax: (1) 760 431 6948 or (800) 650 5115
www.hayhouse.com

Published and distributed in Australia by:
Hay House Australia Ltd, 18/36 Ralph St, Alexandria NSW 2015
Tel: (61) 2 9669 4299; Fax: (61) 2 9669 4144
www.hayhouse.com.au

Published and distributed in the Republic of South Africa by:
Hay House SA (Pty) Ltd, PO Box 990, Witkoppen 2068
Tel/Fax: (27) 11 467 8904
www.hayhouse.co.za

Published and distributed in India by:
Hay House Publishers India, Muskaan Complex, Plot No.3, B-2,
Vasant Kunj, New Delhi 110 070
Tel: (91) 11 4176 1620; Fax: (91) 11 4176 1630
www.hayhouse.co.in

Distributed in Canada by:
Raincoast, 9050 Shaughnessy St, Vancouver BC V6P 6E5
Tel: (1) 604 323 7100; Fax: (1) 604 323 2600

Text © Charlie Morley, 2013

The moral rights of the author have been asserted.

The information given in this book should not be treated as a substitute for professional
medical advice; always consult a medical practitioner. Any use of information in this book is at
the reader's discretion and risk. Neither the author nor the publisher can be held responsible
for any loss, claim or damage arising out of the use, or misuse, of the suggestions made, the
failure to take medical advice or for any material on third party websites.

Interior images: 1, 61, 189 fybe:one

A catalogue record for this book is available from the British Library.

ISBN: 978-1-78180-202-1

Printed and bound in Great Britain by TJ International, Padstow, Cornwall.

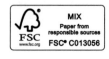

For the dakinis,
the awakened women
to whom I owe so much.

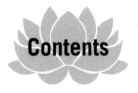

Contents

Part III: Germination

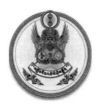

Foreword

Buddhist meditation is ultimately about liberating the mind from illusion and self-deception. To this end it is necessary to train the mind and develop kindness, compassion and wisdom. The dreaming mind is fertile ground for developing these qualities. In the Tibetan tradition, the refined discipline of Dream Yoga has been practised for a thousand years, and as one of the famous Six Yogas of Naropa it is an important element in our intensive four-year retreats at Samye Ling Monastery. The stability of the lucid dream is the foundation of Dream Yoga.

In *Dreams of Awakening*, Charlie Morley is offering a useful, practical synthesis of both Western and Tibetan Buddhist approaches to dream work, and the Western methods of inducing lucid dreams are a significant support for anyone wishing to engage the practice of Dream Yoga in the future.

I am one of Charlie's teachers and have a strong connection with him; through this I have confidence in his honest simplicity and trust his methods. His clarity, humility and humanity make it easier for people to understand his presentation of this deep and important subject of lucid dream, and I am satisfied that people who study this book and attend his courses can trust him. Charlie's approach is particularly valuable because he is offering methods of working with dream and sleep that will help people in societies where relevant methods have until now been lacking.

I recommend this book to anyone who wishes to benefit from living a more awakened life.

Lama Yeshe Losal Rinpoche
Chairman of Rokpa Trust
Abbot of Kagyu Samye Ling
Executive Director of the Holy Isle Project

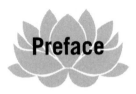

Preface

'I can't get lucid in my dreams... am I a failure?'

Maybe not. Lucidity is not only about the dream dimension, it's about all dimensions – being awake, washing the dishes, falling asleep, daydreaming, waking up and all the rest. So, what is the essential ingredient? Recognition. No matter what is being experienced, *recognition*.

Most of us blunder through our life in a miasma of confusion, driven by unseen urges and desires that leave us feeling unfulfilled, lonely and empty. It's common to feel cut off, out of touch, pointless, because we often only experience a small part of what we are – the superficial part. Many of us sense there is more, but don't know how to reach it. This is frustrating because this 'more' seems to be significant. That's why lucidity is so relevant.

The power of recognition we develop in lucidity training changes our experience of all aspects of life and helps us cut through neurotic confusion to access our inherent potential for insight and wisdom. These qualities are the basis of a happy, free mind that can embark upon the journey to psychological and spiritual growth.

The question is how to do it.

Effective methods for establishing lucidity in dreams have been developed in the West, and Charlie has mastered and added to these. One of his unique innovations has been lucid dreaming retreats involving sleep-ins where participants sleep side by side and get woken up at key times through the night and day. I have been involved with two of these and was struck by how quickly people became lucid in this environment.

Perhaps more important is our realization that the hypnagogic (falling-asleep state) and hypnopompic (waking-up period) are just as significant for learning and growth as lucid dreams. This is good news for people who struggle to get lucid because it means they have alternative areas for training. I suspect these might be more important for the beginner than actual dreams, because they are more accessible, and are places where we can experience a free flow of psychological material we normally suppress – especially the hypnopompic. This seems to have become my speciality and I can sometimes spend hours in this state during the dawn period. The mind is softer then, more relaxed, and is therefore able to embrace powerful emotions it would normally block. This allows an environment where deep insights and integration of disturbing psychological states are possible. These are essential for growth and maturation. It's almost as though a parallel universe opens up to us, enabling swift integration of unresolved psychology that might otherwise take a lifetime. It's also a place where we can be instructed by our deeper wisdom.

This book offers you practical instruction and guidance for developing recognition and increased awareness in many areas of life. It shows you how to expand the magic of lucidity beyond dream into falling asleep, waking up and ultimately living.

Rob Nairn, author of *Living, Dreaming, Dying*

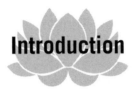

Introduction

In 1881, E.E. Barnard discovered a new galaxy. At the time, it wasn't recognized as a galaxy because the notion of multiple galaxies was deemed ridiculous. There was only one galaxy – ours. The Milky Way was the entire universe. A couple of decades into the 20th century it was finally conceded that there could be up to a dozen galaxies – although many people still thought this impossible. We now know that there are over 100 billion galaxies just in the tiny section of the universe that we know about. From one galaxy to 100 billion galaxies in one lifetime.

By expanding our awareness of the vastness of the universe, scientific enquiry helps us wake up from the slumber of ignorance and open our eyes to the sense of infinity and abundance. And, paradoxically, the mystery deepens.

There is a revolution afoot and it is not restricted to our knowledge of outer space. Just as there are astronauts, so there are oneironauts – intrepid dream explorers following ancient esoteric maps to inner space and finding there a similar vastness, filled with worlds of wonder.

In his book *The Inner Reaches of Outer Space*, the great mythologist Joseph Campbell writes, 'Indeed, the first and most essential service of a mythology is this one, of opening the mind and heart to the utter wonder of all being.'

As we grow older, we seem to lose that sense of recognition. As our responsibilities increase and anxieties gather, we rush headlong into the future while dragging our past behind us. But there's a place where we can still be children and play with epiphanies – in our dreams. Campbell was writing about myths, but he might as well have been writing about our nightly dreams.

'But dreams aren't real' comes the knee-jerk objection – a response that can only come from someone who hasn't experienced a fully lucid dream. When we become lucid in our dreams and learn to stabilize that lucidity, we quickly learn that a lucid dream is as real as waking reality. It's just a reality with different dimensions.

This book will explore those dimensions. Using a three-part structure of Ground, Path and Germination, my aim is to offer a map which, if followed, will allow the recognition of the dream state to become the recognition of our mind's true potential.

After a solid grounding in the history, context and benefits of lucid dreaming within both Western and Buddhist traditions, we'll set off down the path of learning how to be mindfully aware in our dreams and sleep. Then finally we'll explore the germination of the practice, journey into the frontier lands and see just how deep the rabbit hole goes.

Words can't convey the sense of actual participation in this adventure. The journey won't be in reading this book but in where it will inspire you to go. So, let's set off on the road… to dreams of awakening…

PART I
GROUND

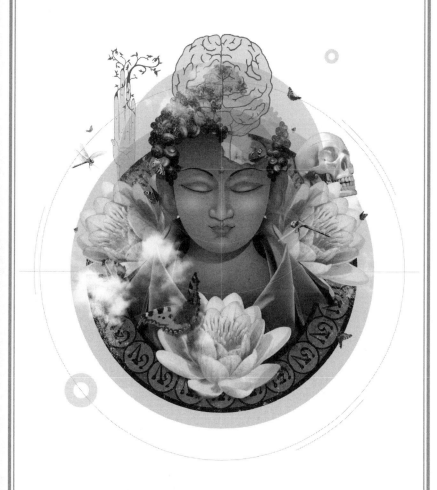

The Basics

'Let us learn to dream, and then we may
perhaps find the truth.'
FRIEDRICH KEKULÉ

Lucid dreaming is both magical and misunderstood in equal measure. That's why it's useful to have a stable ground of understanding before applying the practice. So let's prepare our ground, weed out the facts from the fiction and open our mind to the limitless potential of the field before us.

WHAT IS A LUCID DREAM?

To start by clarifying terms, a lucid dream is a dream in which we are actively aware that we are dreaming as the dream is happening. But don't be deceived by this dry definition. Lucid dreams are commonly described as among the most thrilling experiences to be had. A fully lucid dream is not a hazy, imprecise phantasmagoria, but a full-colour, high-definition and hyper-realistic experience. It can profoundly reconfigure our perceptions of reality.

Lucid dreaming is a form of mind training in which we learn consciously to recognize our dreams as dreams while we are dreaming. As with all forms of mind training, the aim is to be more aware and more awake, to switch off the autopilot and to wake up to life. To dream lucidly is to live lucidly.

The term 'lucid dream' was supposedly coined by Frederick van Eeden, a Dutch psychiatrist, 100 years ago,[1] but is misleading. My workshop participants sometimes describe a particularly intense, vivid dream they have had and ask whether this could be classified as a lucid dream. My answer is always that if you have to ask whether a dream was lucid, it probably wasn't. When you've had a fully lucid dream, you won't be left wondering if it qualified.

To avoid this confusion, some have put forward the alternative term 'conscious dreaming'. But the word 'lucid' originally conveyed the meaning of 'having insight', rather than describing the perceptual quality of the experience. It is this element of insight that is the cornerstone of the lucid dream. In fact, it reveals the profound potential of the mind in a way that few other states of consciousness can, because through lucid dreaming we become aware of awareness itself.

This awakening of awareness within the dream state is not accompanied by any physiological awakening. To all outward appearances, we are still sound asleep and 'unconscious', yet internally, in our dreaming mind, it could be said that we are wide awake. Van Eeden commented, 'In lucid dreams the sleeper remembers his daily life [and] reaches a state of perfect awareness... Yet the sleep is undisturbed, deep and refreshing.'[2]

It seems a contradiction to be both aware and asleep at the same time, and this neurological paradox means that it was only in the late 1970s that lucid dreaming came to be verified by Western scientific means.

More recently, studies from Frankfurt University's neurological clinic and the Max Planck Institute of Psychiatry have found that specific alterations to brain physiology appear once a dreamer becomes lucid. Using brain-imaging technology such as magnetic resonance tomography and EEG, scientists can now pinpoint the actual 'Aha! I'm dreaming!' moment of lucid awareness and its neurophysiological correlates. The researchers concluded that 'lucid dreaming constitutes a hybrid state of consciousness with definable and measurable differences from the waking state and from the REM [rapid eye movement] dream state'.[3] They discovered that when lucid consciousness was attained within the dream, activity in areas associated with self-assessment and self-perception increased markedly within seconds.[4] This means the apparent paradox of being both aware and asleep, which had previously caused a lot of resistance and scepticism from the scientific establishment, was simply a failure to understand how two distinct brain regions could be activated simultaneously.

The thing that surprises most first-time lucid dreamers is the fact that fully lucid dreams are not very dreamy at all. The lucid dream state both looks and feels real. It is a meticulously intricate mental construct that often appears as realistic as our waking reality. It may, in fact, seem so real that we come to question our perceptions of waking reality and stand in awe of the creative aptitude of the human mind. Since I started training, I've had hundreds of lucid dreams and yet am still struck by the infinite potential of lucid dreaming and its capacity to facilitate entire dimensions of 'reality' within our own minds. The lucid dream environment is often so meticulously realistic that some new lucid dreamers come to the audacious conclusion that it can't be a dream at all and they must have travelled to another dimension. And indeed they have – a dimension within their own mind.

Does this mean lucid dreamers stand to lose touch with reality? No, in fact quite the opposite – once we can penetrate the persuasive reality of the dreamscape and know it as an illusion, we become better equipped to recognize self-deception in the waking state. This makes us more grounded and more aware.

If you haven't had a lucid dream yet, or are still unsure as to what one actually constitutes, take a moment now to check out some of the lucid dreams in the appendices at the back of this book. Please do take a moment to do this.*

Essentially, during a lucid dream the mind is creating an incredibly detailed three-dimensional projection to form the functional reality of the dreamscape, while another part of the mind is consciously interacting with this projection in real time. So, in a lucid dream we are both the creator and the created, the projector and the projected.

This mind-boggling process reveals the infinite potential of the brain in a way few other states of consciousness can, because through lucid dreaming we become conscious within our unconscious. This opens up the possibility of directly interacting with psychological aspects and archetypes at a seemingly tangible level.

My friend the lucid dreaming expert Robert Waggoner once told me, 'Lucid dreaming helps us to see the magic that already exists.' It's true: while we are learning to see through illusion, lucid dreaming nonetheless gives us a tangible experience of the magic of the dream state.

In a fully lucid dream, the quality of cognitive awareness allows us to interact directly with the dream and to influence it. Given enough lucidity, we can experience a dream with exactly the same reflective awareness as when we are awake. We know that we are actually asleep in our bed, we remember what we had planned to do once lucid and we know that we are moving around our own psyche.

---

* Not everybody likes to read through other people's lucid dreams (which is why I haven't included any in the main body of the text), but there are over 20 of my own in the appendices for those that do.

Lucid dreaming is not easy to master, but it is undeniably one of the most exciting and rewarding practices we may ever engage in, with a wealth of both psychological and spiritual benefits. Within the framework of Mindfulness of Dream & Sleep (more about that later), it's a completely safe practice, open to all ages and abilities, offering a unique insight into our own psychology.

In a letter to a mourning friend Albert Einstein once wrote, 'A human being… experiences himself, his thoughts and feelings as something separated from the rest – a kind of optical delusion of his consciousness… To try to overcome this delusion is the way to attain true peace of mind.'[5]

Through lucid dreaming we can overcome this delusion as we experience a fully realistic 'reality' which may seem separate from us, but which we know we are dreaming into existence and is actually within us. Thus we are introduced, in visceral fashion, to the radical notion that duality may be a delusion. In a lucid dream we are one with everything, because we *are* everything. This experience can help dissolve our sense of isolation in the waking state, allowing us finally to wake up to the Oneness on which Einstein and the mystics of the ages have been so eloquent.

WHAT IS THE LUCIDITY SPECTRUM?

Dreaming is not as clear-cut as just 'lucid' or 'non-lucid'. There is, rather, a lucidity spectrum based on the degrees of awareness within the dream, ranging from a suspicion that we might be dreaming to fully conscious reflective awareness.

I've identified four main levels of lucidity, although this is a very basic system of categorization and it's not necessary to stick to it rigidly. Our transition through the spectrum is not always a linear one either, and although Level 1 may often lead to Level 2 and so on, it is also common to find ourselves at Level 3 or 4 straightaway, thanks to a sudden burst of awareness.

Level 1: Pre-lucid

'Pre-lucid' is a term coined by lucid dream researcher Celia Green to describe the state of mind in which we critically question the reality of the dream. Although this experience can lead straight to lucidity, it's often a state that beginner lucid dreamers may visit frustratingly frequently without becoming lucid.

In the pre-lucid state, suspicions arise that we might be dreaming, usually after we have become aware of some bizarre dream anomaly. For example, we are pre-lucid if we find ourselves thinking, *Hang on, I don't usually go out in public in my underwear… Could I be dreaming?*

Level 2: Semi-lucid

Here we experience the 'Aha!' moment of lucid awareness but then slip back and forth between lucidity and non-lucidity. We may be lucid one moment, then become distracted by the dream and slip back into non-lucidity.

More commonly, the initial 'lucidity flash' can be so exciting that we wake ourselves up. *Hang on, I don't usually go out in public in my underwear… Could I be dreaming?* soon becomes *Oh wow! I actually am dreaming! This is so exciting! I can't wait to try to…* and then we find ourselves awake in our bed. In fact, for some beginners this initial over-excitability means that their first few lucid dreams may only last a matter of seconds before they wake up. (We'll look at ways to avoid this in Part II.)

Level 3: Fully Lucid

This is the state of fully conscious reflective awareness within the dream, coupled with volitional interaction with the dreamscape and dream characters.

Here we are fully aware that we're dreaming and can begin to influence the dreamscape and narrative of the dream by engaging in whatever activity we want to do. With full lucidity, we can maintain awareness for the entirety of the dream period, which may be an hour or more in length.

Many believe this is the highest possible level of lucidity. I disagree – there is a deeper level.

Level 4: Super-lucid

This is a term borrowed from Robert Waggoner to describe the state in which we have a level of awareness that surpasses full lucidity, due to an experience of partial non-dual awareness.

What does this mean? The fundamental difference between 'fully lucid' and 'super-lucid' rests on a subtle but profound shift of perception. Most of us experiencing a fully lucid dream will interact with the dream as if it is waking reality. For example, we might use a door to get from one room to another or fly through the air to travel to a new place. In a super-lucid dream, however, we'll just walk straight through the wall or instantly appear somewhere at will rather than travel there. While super-lucid, we base all our actions upon the realization that everything in the dream is a creation of the mind, without slipping back into the dualistic interactions of lower-level full lucidity.*

Witnessing Dream

This type of dream falls within the lucidity spectrum but doesn't quite fit into any of the four levels described above. We experience a witnessing dream from a gentle non-preferential perspective, fully aware that we are dreaming but without any desire to influence or interact with the dream. Instead we allow it to unfold on its own, often as though we are watching it on a movie screen.

---

* A super-lucid dream is, for many people, an experience approaching non-dual awareness in which the clarity of mind is so strong that it may temporarily dissolve the dreamer's sense of self.

Witnessing dreams can happen spontaneously but are a common product of prolonged meditation – the meditator effectively carries the daytime's quiet non-preferential mindfulness into the night.

Don't worry too much about the different levels of lucidity. I've included the lucidity spectrum here more as a way to explore the nature of lucidity rather than to make it a cornerstone of the practice.

DOES LUCID DREAMING MEAN WE'RE CONTROLLING OUR DREAMS?

Many books and websites promise the ability to 'control your dreams through lucid dreaming', but this is an ill-advised – and arguably impossible – aim. Although it's true that with training an advanced practitioner can gain a remarkable level of volitional influence over many aspects of their subjective experience, there is always a much larger aspect of mind creating the majority of the dream.

Once lucid, it is of course natural to want to exert our will. One of the most popular lucid dream activities seems to be flying, so let's work with that example. Say you become lucid and choose to fly into the sky. Raise your fist to the sky and you're off like Superman. You're controlling the dream, right? Wrong.

Even in a lucid dream in which you're flying through the air controlling your elevation and velocity at will, there is still a much larger aspect of mind creating and managing the dream landscape that you're flying over and the dream sky that you're flying in. Did you choose to have those dream characters walking the streets below you? You may be controlling your subjective experience of the localized dreamscape, but there is something much more powerful directing everything else.

Waggoner says, 'No sailor controls the sea. Similarly, no lucid dreamer controls the dream.'[6] It would be an arrogant sailor who believed that they were controlling the awesome power of the sea, and it's just the same with our dreams. I didn't always believe this, though. Through a lot of intensive training, I once reached a level of lucidity in which I would change the entire dreamscape just because I could, silence dream characters to show them I was boss and forcefully reject new lines of narrative in favour of my own. I thought that finally, after years of practice, I had mastered full control over my dreams, but in fact I was disregarding the music of the dreaming mind and forcefully dancing to my own beat, totally out of synch with what the dream was trying to offer. These attempts would invariably lead to a loving but firm slap from the motherly dreaming mind, either through an inexplicable loss of lucid control or a bombardment of nightmarish shadow material.

Once I began to relinquish the excessive control I had been exercising, something strange happened – I started to have more volitional influence within my lucid dreams, not less. It was as if once I had shifted my motivation from *control* to *co-creation*, the dreaming mind responded positively by giving me more lucid capacity.

A sailor may grow to know the sea so well that he sails *as if* he were in control. So, too, we can come to sail upon the ocean of our dreaming mind.

ARE WE MESSING WITH THE UNCONSCIOUS?

Another concern we should address at the outset is the fear that by lucid dreaming we may somehow be interfering with the integrity of the unconscious by bringing awareness into an area of our mind that normally seems to function autonomously. Thankfully, this fear is groundless.

Rather than lucid dreaming polluting the pure message from the deeper part of ourselves, it actually allows that message to be heeded more easily, which I believe is exactly what the unconscious mind wants. The unconscious actually enjoys lucidity, because finally a line of direct communication is being set up between it and the conscious mind and it 'takes joy in dealing with greater awareness and greater consciousness'.[7] Finally, it can talk to us face to face.

With every dream, the unconscious mind is offering us a hand of friendship. But far too often this is an offering we ignore, either by not remembering our dreams or by failing to acknowledge their value. Once we become lucidly aware within the dream, however, we are extending a hand towards the unconscious mind and finally making friends with it.

As Rob Preece says in *The Psychology of Buddhist Tantra*, 'When we are willing to take the psyche seriously, and listen to its symbolic expression, we can gain greater clarity and insight into the forces that influence us. We will no longer be victims of the unconscious.'[8]

This is one of the core benefits of lucid dreaming: making friends with ourselves. We don't get lucid so we can try and control the unconscious mind or boss it about, we get lucid so that we can make friends with it, commune with it and finally start listening to it.

As with any friendship, we have to learn to accept our new friend on equal terms, not censoring or arguing with them, but listening to them with an open heart. This is the most important friendship we may ever have, and it is a friendship that will spill over into our waking state, too, in sudden bursts of creativity or spontaneous insights which let us know our new friend is always with us – even when we're not dreaming.

Although this friendship may be on equal terms, the unconscious has been running the dream state for much longer than we've been having lucid dreams and so it will always be the stronger force. We're not talking about taking some drug that compels the unconscious mind to accommodate lucid awareness, but a process by which the dreaming mind opens the door and allows lucidity into its domain.* This means that if it doesn't like what we're doing in the lucid dream it will simply block our attempts to do whatever it is, so to think that we can 'mess with the unconscious' just because we are lucid is to ascribe an inflated degree of influence to our conscious mind.

CAN ANYONE DO IT?

The good news is that anybody can learn to lucid dream. In fact, we don't even really need to learn, we just need to remember. This is because we've all been great lucid dreamers in the past. Every child is a lucid dreamer – the adult's task is merely to relearn the skill.

Children naturally have lucid dreams.[9] Why? I believe it is connected to creativity. Children are naturally right-brain dominant, meaning they are attuned to the creative, imaginative, intuitive side of their brain. But as they grow up, they switch sides to the more logical, calculating, left-brain dominance of adulthood. Dreaming is an almost entirely right-brain activity, so it seems that once we lose our connection to the creativity of our brain's right hemisphere, we also lose the connection to our dreams – and our natural ability to become lucid within them. In short, we forget how to lucid dream when we forget how to be children. Artistic adults such as actors, musicians and artists, however, often retain their right-brain inclination, which is why they also seem to have spontaneous lucid dreams more often than other people.

---

* We have about five dream periods each night, so even if we have one lucid dream every night, there are still four other dream periods in which our unconscious mind can run wild and free.

So, lucid dreaming is a perfectly natural state of mind and we can regain it. The Buddha once said, 'It doesn't matter how long you have forgotten, only how soon you remember.' So don't worry how long it has been since you last had a lucid dream – let's just concentrate on remembering how to do it again. The fact is, if you dream, you can lucid dream – it just takes some practice.

Throughout this book I quote research studies from many different sleep laboratories, but the best 'sleep lab' we have is the one in our own dreaming mind, a lab to which we have access every night.

When I was a teenager, the free accessibility of lucid dreaming was one of its real selling points for me. There was no equipment to be bought, no initiation to be done, no club to join. The only commodities required were sleep and determination. And the great thing about dream work, compared to other mind-training tools, is that hardly a 24-hour period goes by without the opportunity to practise. Whether you are a nightshift worker snoozing in the afternoon, a student sleeping till lunchtime or a pensioner dozing during the day, there is always time for lucid dreaming.

As with all skills, some people may find it easier than others. It seems that having two X chromosomes can help, as women report more lucid dreams and have better dream recall than men, but essentially lucid dreaming is open to everyone. Teenagers and people under the age of 30 have longer dream periods and thus slightly more opportunity to practise, but unless you have a strong motivation to become lucid, it doesn't matter how much dream time you have. I've taught everyone from 12-year-olds to 70-year-olds and the defining characteristic of success is motivation, not age.

A lot of the lucid dreaming workshops and retreats that I run take place at Buddhist centres and I have found that practising meditators have a much higher rate of lucid dreams than non-meditators, with some of them having spontaneous lucid dreams on a weekly basis. This is because mindful awareness during the day directly translates into mindful awareness during dreams. In fact one of the original lucid dream induction techniques (and one that we will learn more about in Part II) is mindfulness meditation.

If meditation seems a bit too static for you, then it seems that getting down on the dance floor might work just as well. Before teaching lucid dreaming, I spent many years working in the world of professional breakdancing and I noticed that many of my dancer friends found lucid dreaming remarkably easy. Was it all that spinning on their head that did it? Perhaps – dream researcher Jayne Gackenbach says that due to the link between the vestibular system of balance found in the inner ear and the production of eye movements during dreams, people who have good physical body balance (such as breakdancers) are often good at lucid dreaming.[10] Another finding Gackenbach came up with is one of my personal favourites: apparently lucid dreamers are 'often people who lean towards an androgynous temperament and those who are willing to take internal risks such as trying shamanic drumming'.[11]

So it seems that if you are an artistic, mindful, breakdancing female shamanic-drumming teenager then you might find lucid dreaming a bit easier than the rest of us. But if you are none of the above, not to worry – we can all learn how to lucid dream. And in Part II I'll show you how.

WHAT IS MINDFULNESS OF DREAM & SLEEP?

Mindfulness of Dream & Sleep is a holistic approach to lucid dreaming and conscious sleeping that I have created with Buddhist meditation teacher, Rob Nairn. This new approach is not just about learning how to lucid dream; rather, it is about how to use all areas of falling asleep, dreaming and waking up for spiritual and psychological growth.

Mindfulness of Dream & Sleep is comprised of three main practices: mindfulness meditation, lucid dream training from both the Western and Tibetan Buddhist traditions and conscious sleeping techniques called 'hypnagogic and hypnopompic mindfulness'. Don't fret about the odd names for now – all will be clarified later on. Our hope is that by combining Western and Eastern techniques we can bridge the gap between the often superficial scope of Western lucid dreaming practices and the often inaccessible Tibetan dream yoga practices. Mindfulness of Dream & Sleep is for people who want to go beyond lucid dreaming into something much deeper.

Mindfulness of Dream & Sleep is essentially about bringing mindful awareness into all stages of our sleep cycle, allowing us to make use of the full 30 years we spend asleep, rather than just the six years we spend dreaming. By developing our training across all phases of sleep, rather than just within the lucid dream state, we can offer a far more holistic and wide-ranging system with benefits that extend well beyond our dream world into our waking life.

Much like lucid dreaming, Mindfulness of Dream & Sleep may sound like a paradox, because we are so accustomed to thinking of dream and sleep as unmindful processes. However, it is possible to be aware during most periods of dream and sleep, and this awareness will paradoxically lead to more refreshing and beneficial sleep.

The ultimate aim is to allow mindful awareness to gently infuse all stages of our sleep cycle. This leads to a deep deconditioning process that will also permeate our waking state, allowing us to 'wake up' to life with more awareness and to live as we dream: lucidly.

2

Where Science and Spirituality Meet

'The history of the world is none other than the
progress of the consciousness of freedom.'
<small>HEGEL</small>

It's just gone 8 a.m. on a rainy spring morning at Hull University, 1975. Psychologist Keith Hearne is hunched over a recording apparatus charting the eye movements, muscle tone and EEG brain activity of his sleeping subject, a 37-year-old lucid dreamer named Alan Worsley. Although he doesn't know it yet, Worsley is about to make history.

When Hearne decided to tackle the scientific verification of lucid dreaming, the concept was still scoffed at by the scientific community as being a 'paradoxical impossibility'. Regardless of thousands of years of first-hand reports and an entire arena of Buddhist teachings on the subject, most sleep and dream researchers considered the idea of conscious awareness within dreams a flaky new-age delusion.

Hearne's contemporaries realized that the only way to verify lucid dreaming scientifically would be to get data that proved two things simultaneously: first, that the dreamer was dreaming and not partially awake; second, that the dreamer was consciously signalling to the outside world from within the dream world. But how to send such a signal without waking up? During dreaming sleep the body is paralysed – with the exception of the respiratory system and the eyes. Hearne had a hunch that the eyes could be used to send that all-important signal.

Before falling asleep, Worsley was instructed to try to become lucid and then engage in a set of smooth horizontal eye movements (very different from the random flitting and rolling of REM sleep). These signals would then be picked up by the eye-movement recorders in the lab, while the EEG machine would keep track of his brain activity.

The night passed with little success, but in the final hour of Worsley's sleep cycle his periods of REM became more frequent. Hearne had been watching Worsley dreaming for about half an hour when something remarkable happened.

'Suddenly, out of the jumbled, senseless to's and fro's of the two eye-movement recording channels, a regular set of large zigzags appeared on the chart,' Hearne recalls in his book *The Dream Machine*. 'Instantly I was alert and felt the greatest exhilaration upon realizing that I was observing the first ever deliberate signals sent from within the dream to the outside world.'[1] The 'impossible' had finally been proved.

Around the same time that Hearne was pioneering the scientific verification of lucid dreaming in the UK, in the USA a bright young lucid dreamer was starting work on his PhD in psychophysiology at Stanford University in California. This prodigal dreamer was Stephen LaBerge, a name that would become synonymous with lucid dreaming across the globe. Working at Stanford, LaBerge set out to prove for the first time in history the existence of lucid dreaming – or so he thought.

How could he not have known about Hearne's results? Although Hearne did deliver a paper to a conference on behavioural sciences in 1977, then published his PhD thesis a year later, 'the scientific establishment resisted accepting his results'.[2] The upshot was that his proof was simply never widely circulated, peer-reviewed or disseminated across the Atlantic. When LaBerge finally got similar results using similar methods, he naturally believed that he had broken new ground. This proved a useful illusion, as it fed his determination to spread the news when all the top journals (including the esteemed *Science*) refused to publish his research. Eventually, in 1981, a lesser-known scientific journal, *Perceptual and Motor Skills*, published his findings.[3] This, along with a primetime lecture spot at the Association for the Psychophysiological Study of Sleep's annual conference, was the start of an epic career that would make LaBerge the pioneer of lucid dreaming in the West.

LaBerge's passion for the subject and his notable aptitude both for lucid dreaming and for teaching it to others have relegated much of Hearne's impeccable research to a footnote in the history books. However, without LaBerge's tireless work over the last three decades in both the public and scientific spheres, lucid dreaming books might still be on the back shelf next to texts on alien abduction and Victorian superstition. To both Hearne and LaBerge, we would do well to doff our hats.

BEYOND THE IMAGINATION

Since those initial experiments in the days of disco, scientific research into lucid dreaming has thrown up scores of weird and wonderful new discoveries, with one conclusion and its implications standing out from the rest.

Using EEG machines, eye-movement and muscle-tone monitors, with experiments that involved activities like singing*

---

* Interestingly, the first song to be sung in the lucid dream state by LaBerge's research team was 'Life is but a Dream'.

and mental arithmetic within the actual lucid dream state, it was discovered that lucid dream actions elicited the exact same neurological responses as actions performed while awake. Further research found that the same correlations existed for a whole range of lucid dream activities, such as holding the breath, estimating time (lucid dream time and waking time feeling roughly the same) and even sexual function.

The implications are huge – our neurological system doesn't differentiate between waking and lucid dream experiences. In other words, for our brain, there is no discernible difference between lucid dreams and waking life. Dreaming lucidly about doing something is not like imagining it – it's like actually doing it.

The potential benefits of this finding are profound. In the waking state, if we imagine happy scenarios, we usually only induce a slight increase in neurologically measurable happiness. In the lucid dream state, however, if we engage in an activity that bring us joy and happiness (whether it's flying, swimming with dolphins or playing bass for the Beatles), the synapses in the parts of the brain associated with happiness light up and release feel-good chemicals in exactly the same way as if we were experiencing these activities while awake. To our psychophysical system, a lucid dream isn't just a visualization – it's a reality.

This revelation opens up a whole arena for psychological healing and growth. For example, neural pathways can be strengthened and created in our lucid dreams just as they can while we are awake due to the function of neuroplasticity.* So, lucid dreamers who consciously engage in beneficial activities within their dreams are creating and strengthening beneficial neural pathways, which will then become habitually engaged in the waking state. This means that we can *learn* in our lucid dreams.

---

* Neuroplasticity describes the brain's ability to rewire itself as part of a never-ending capacity for change. It shows us that old dogs *can* learn new tricks, and that it's never too late to learn a new skill.

There is one tradition that learned of the benefits of lucid dream work a long time ago…

BUDDHA: THE MAN WHO WOKE UP

About 2,500 years ago, five centuries before Jesus, a young Sakyan prince in the foothills of the Himalayas became the original rich-kid dropout. His name was Siddhartha Gautama. At the age of 29, after a palatial life of luxury during which he had been kept blissfully ignorant of the suffering of the world, he decided to radically change both his lifestyle and his mind. He wanted to wake up.

Siddhartha's slumber was first disturbed when he left his upper-class bubble and saw how poor people lived – with the pains of old age, sickness and death. On a trip out of his gated kingdom, he also saw a wandering holy man, a sight that left an indelible impression on him. Much like celebrities nowadays who do aid work in Africa and come back changed by their experiences, Siddhartha was deeply affected by what he saw when he left the palace grounds. Rather than set up a rock concert to raise money for charity, he decided to focus on the root of the problem: innate human suffering and how to overcome it.

Without telling anybody except his assistant, Siddhartha slipped out from the palace one night, leaving his lavish lifestyle behind to go and live as a mendicant monk. For years he wandered India, learning from some of the greatest meditation masters of his time. Unsatisfied with mental states of deep spiritual absorption, he eventually focused on practising radical asceticism in an attempt to tame the mind through mortification of the body. Despite some benefits, this approach nearly killed him, and so, considering the hedonism of his princely upbringing and the extreme asceticism that nearly ended his life, he finally decided to pioneer a 'middle way' between these extremes.

At the age of 35, he left his fellow ascetics and went to a place now called Bodh Gaya, where he sat down under a tree and vowed not to rise until he had achieved total spiritual awakening. A full 49 days of solid meditation later, he arose from his seat under the tree as the Awakened One: the Buddha. He had finally 'woken up' fully from the sleep of ignorance and soon he would begin to teach others how to wake up, too.

Buddhist scholar Stephen Batchelor says: 'What happened to the Buddha beneath that tree is comparable, or is similar to, the experience that each of us has every morning when the alarm goes off and we wake up.'[4] The moment we wake up each morning, we gain a lucid insight – what we have taken as real has actually been a dream, an intricate illusion. This is what happened to the Buddha, the only difference being that whereas we wake from dreams to waking reality, he woke from waking reality to ultimate reality.

BUDDHISM: TEACHINGS ON HOW TO WAKE UP

I started practising Buddhism when I was 19. Since then I have received teachings from some of the leading meditation masters and most esteemed gurus on the planet. What knowledge do I have to show for it? Very little. What enlightened qualities do I now possess? None. So what do I have to show for over a decade of mind exploration? I am much friendlier than I used to be.

Buddhism is all about friendliness. Unconditional friendliness towards yourself and towards others. Unconditional friendliness towards pain and towards happiness, towards joy and towards despair. For me, that's the essence of the Buddha's teachings – unconditional friendliness towards everything.

We can sum up the Buddha's message as: 'Do no harm, be kind and tame your mind.' A Buddhist practitioner tries to engage in as many forms of wise, loving, compassionate action as possible, while avoiding actions that do harm to oneself or others.

Buddhism won't make you more popular or more attractive but what it can do is to 'help you cut through your confusion and your neuroses. Buddhism can help you understand yourself.'[5]

This practical self-understanding is a recurring theme throughout the teachings, as are compassion and wisdom. Compassion without wisdom becomes blind sentimentality, which can often do more harm than good, but when coupled with insightful wisdom, it can be applied in a way that really works. Wisdom is the cultivation of insight into how things really are and the Buddha taught that one of the best ways to cultivate this insight was through meditation.

Meditation is a system of relaxed reflection and mind training that leads to awareness and insight. Meditating and reflecting bring us into direct contact with what is happening with our inner environment, so that we come to know ourselves better. And the better we know ourselves, the better equipped we are to help others.

The Buddha didn't set out to found a religion or to convert people to a belief – he simply taught a system of ethics, compassion and loving kindness towards all beings, which aimed to help people wake up to their own enlightened nature. He said, 'Don't blindly believe what I say. Find out for yourself what is true, what is real.' His teaching tools were meditation techniques that tamed the selfish mind and practical guidelines on how to live joyfully with wisdom and compassion. These tools are as applicable today as they were 2,500 years ago, and in fact the more modern science discovers about the nature of the mind, the more the Buddha's teachings ring true. Eventually they became 'Buddhism' – both a religion and a way of life that has spread around the globe.

There are three main schools of Buddhism: Theravada (the teachings of the elders), Mahayana (the greater vehicle) and

Vajrayana (the diamond vehicle). We will focus primarily on the Vajrayana, which flourished mainly in Tibet and was developed with two unique aims in mind: enlightenment within one lifetime and 24-hour spiritual practice.

DREAMING ON THE ROOF OF THE WORLD

Dreams have played a central role in Buddhism ever since the 'conception dream' of the Buddha's mother, Maya. In fact, the notion of conscious dreaming was put forth by the Buddha himself. In the *Pali Vinaya*, the original rulebook for monks and nuns, the Buddha actually instructs his followers to fall asleep in a state of mindfulness as a way to prevent 'seeing a bad dream' or 'waking unhappily'.[6] So it seems that the healing potential of mindful sleeping goes right back to the source.

However, the first integrated system of lucid dream work would only be created well over 1,000 years later, when Vajrayana Buddhism found its way into Tibet. There it encountered an indigenous form of mysticism called Bön, which had a long history of shamanic dream practices.

Tibetan Buddhism thus developed out of a synthesis of this indigenous shamanic religion and Vajrayana Buddhist teachings. Both of these traditions practised dream work, so it's not surprising that in Tibetan Buddhism we find dreams playing such an important role.

Tibetan folklore and the biographies of Buddhist saints are littered with references to dreams. In Tibetan Buddhism itself, dreams are indispensably significant insofar as they are used to find reincarnated masters, to predict future events and as mediums through which to receive spiritual teachings. The recognition of their significance led to the development of a systematic path of practice called dream yoga.

Tibetan Dream Yoga

It would be easy to say that dream yoga was a Tibetan Buddhist form of lucid dreaming, but that would also be lazy and inaccurate. Dream yoga is a collection of transformational lucid dreaming, conscious sleeping and what in the West we refer to as out-of-body experience practices aimed at spiritual growth and mind training. Lucid dreaming may form the foundation of dream yoga, but through the use of advanced tantric energy work, visualizations of Tibetan iconography and the integration of psycho-spiritual archetypes or *yidams*, dream yoga goes way beyond our Western notion of lucid dreaming.

If we translate the Sanskrit word *yoga* as meaning 'union', we get a clue as to what dream yoga is about: the union of consciousness within the dream state. It is a yoga of the mind that uses advanced lucid dreaming methods to utilize sleep on the path to spiritual awakening.

Within Buddhism, illusion and ignorance* are seen as two of the most unbeneficial mind states and there are thousands of practices that aim to transmute them. One of these is dream yoga. Once we're fully lucid in a dream, ignorance is challenged as we recognize that what we thought was real is in fact not real. At the same time, illusion is shattered as we recognize that the entire dreamscape is formed from a mental projection.

As ignorance and illusion dissolve, two highly beneficial states of mind can arise in their place: insight and wisdom. Insight arises as we see clearly that we are dreaming, and wisdom dawns as we understand that our mind is creating our experience. Through dream yoga we can transmute ignorance and illusion while generating wisdom and insight, all while we're sound asleep.

---

* Within Buddhism, ignorance doesn't mean stupidity. It means 'not knowing what really is'. So, a non-lucid dream is a dream of ignorance because we think it's real and don't know that it's a dream.

In some lineages, dream yoga was reserved for those on a three-year retreat and was only taught as part of the famous Six Yogas of Naropa.* These days, however, some of the veils of secrecy have been lifted, allowing it to become a practice that allows dedicated practitioners to extend meditative awareness throughout sleep and dreams, and subsequently throughout death and dying as well. Dreams and death are closely linked in Tibetan Buddhism, as we will explore throughout this book.

The Dalai Lama has said, 'Dream yoga can be practised by both Buddhists and non-Buddhists alike,'[7] and that through dream yoga the lucid dreamer can now engage in spiritual practice while they sleep. So, I encourage you not to feel excluded from this esoteric-sounding practice just because you're not a Buddhist. Although some of the advanced dream yoga techniques should only be engaged in under the guidance of a qualified teacher, there are many techniques that can be practised on your own. We will explore some of these in Part II. Ultimately, it is the motivation behind dream yoga that is the most important aspect of all, fuelling the use of lucid dreaming as a path to spiritual development.

Bardo: The Place in Between

Bardo means 'place in between' and is used to describe any transitional state of existence. Just as dream is the *bardo* between falling asleep and waking up, life is the *bardo* between birth and death. However, what I want to focus on now is the after-death *bardo*, which describes the intermediate states between death and rebirth.

In the Buddhist tradition, sleep is not just a metaphor for death, as it is in the West; it is actually the prime training ground

---

* Naropa was a 10th-century *mahasiddha* who founded the Karma Kagyu school of Tibetan Buddhism. The Six Yogas of Naropa are a series of advanced tantric practices designed to bring the practitioner to full spiritual realization within one lifetime.

for death. Why? Because the after-death *bardo* state is said to be dreamlike in nature. So, it is believed that if we gain mastery over the mind of dreams then we will also have mastery over the mind of death. If we can fall asleep consciously and then recognize our dreams as dreams, we may also be able to die consciously and recognize the after-death *bardo* state. It's said that if practitioners can become fully lucid within the death and after-death *bardo* states, then they can recognize the nature of their mind and have the potential to reach full spiritual awakening.

The practices of lucid dreaming and dream yoga are not only intended to train the practitioner to recognize the after-death *bardo*, but also to train them how to become lucid in their waking state. This lucid awakening within the shared dream of life is exactly what transformed Siddhartha Gautama into the Buddha. This is an awakening that is possible for us all.

3

Why Do We Dream?

'Dreams are the touchstones of our character.'
HENRY DAVID THOREAU

Why do we dream? One might as well ask, why do we live? Nobody knows for sure, but it is a question worth asking and there are three schools of thought that offer some interesting perspectives on the matter: neuroscience, analytical psychology and Tibetan Buddhism.

THE PERSPECTIVE OF NEUROSCIENCE

During dreaming, the mind is projecting dynamic three-dimensional fully operational worlds into which the dreamer is placed. This is a highly active neurological process that actually requires more brain activity and cerebral blood flow than everyday wakefulness. The dreaming brain is not resting, it is working flat out to maintain the intricate projection of our dreaming reality, a projection often so realistic that most of us accept it as real every time we enter it. For most of us it is only upon waking that we realize our folly and distinguish waking reality from that seemingly valid dream reality.

According to some modern brain scientists, the multi-sensory experience of dreaming occurs as a result of chemical changes within the brain as it enters certain phases of sleep. Although neuroscience recognizes that everybody dreams,* it does not recognize the source as being the unconscious mind as such – it regards dreaming as purely chemical. Neurologically, when the brain enters REM sleep, there is a notable change in brain chemistry in which the cells that modulate functions of memory and reflective thought are turned off, meaning that the dreaming brain finds it almost impossible to direct its thoughts, engage in analytical problem-solving or remember its activities.

As these chemical changes occur, the brain begins to create internal hallucinatory realities. Our data-processing routes also shift from logical thought-processing to associative thought-processing, which is why dreams can seem so illogical and bizarre. On top of this, the limbic system, which mediates fear and emotion, shows increased activity, reflecting the intense emotionality of many dreams.**

For most neuroscientists, looking through the prism of evolution, the main purpose of dreaming is 'to facilitate the consolidation and advancement of procedural learning'[1] and to update our memories in such a way that they aid our survival by allowing our mind to replay and learn from certain active and emotional dream scenarios. We dream so that we can digest the day's events and work through new memories, which helps to update our mind with all the latest beneficial sensory input.

One of the most recognizable ways in which dreams aid our survival is through a sense of constant movement. Whether it's travelling somewhere, searching for something or running away

---

* Apart from people who have suffered damage to the multimodal sensory cortex due to a stroke or head injury, everybody dreams, even if not everybody remembers doing so.

** Interestingly, the limbic system does not mature quite like the rest of the brain, so when somebody pushes certain emotional buttons we may react as though we were a four-year-old, even as an adult.

from someone, most people tend to have dreams dominated by movement. Don't believe me? Take a moment and try to remember a dream in which you were sitting completely still…

It is theorized that the dynamic engagement of some movement systems, such as sexual movement, fighting and fleeing, are experienced in dreams to refresh and revise these aids for our survival. Making love and making war are two activities deemed so seemingly important to our brain that we cannot escape them, even in our dreams.

So, it might appear that dreaming is all down to brain chemicals and helping us keep our place on the evolutionary ladder. That's what some neuroscientists think, anyway. But before you make up your own mind, let's lend the psychologists an ear.

'TELL ME YOUR DREAMS'

Sigmund Freud, the father of psychoanalysis and author of *The Interpretation of Dreams*, believed that dreaming was concerned with 'wish fulfilment' and that sexuality was the predominant unconscious force in dreams, as in waking life. However, one of his closest acolytes disagreed: Carl Gustav Jung felt that Freud had merely scratched the surface, and came to believe that the sexual symbolism in dreams was often merely another façade, obscuring deeper, non-sexual, spiritual meanings and psychic functions.

Both Jung and Freud believed that dreams were sourced from our unconscious mind: 'The human mind is divided into two parts, the conscious and the unconscious, with the unconscious being by far the larger of the two.'[2]

The unconscious contains huge stores of information, to which in the waking state the conscious mind has very limited access. It is the unconscious that is revealed in our dreams; so, by recalling our dreams, we enable our conscious mind to view the contents of the unconscious mind.* For Jung, certain dream content was even transpersonal, sourced from a vast storehouse of ancient human experience, containing themes and images found cross-culturally throughout history. This observation led to his concept of the 'collective unconscious', and he argued that dream symbols could also point beyond the personal and into the realm of this depository of human experience.

Today, analytical psychology's perspective on dreaming is based largely on Jung's theories. In his book *Dreams*, Jung held that dreams were fragments of 'involuntary psychic activity', just conscious enough to be memorable in the waking state. He also agreed with Freud that they could often reveal repressed feelings in an uncensored fashion, as well as play a compensatory role and so function as wish-fulfilment. Being fundamentally irrational, dreams were, he believed, hard for the conscious mind to comprehend. They weren't subject to the logic or censorship of waking consciousness and so by dreaming our mind was 'seeking to establish balance within the psyche and to promote psychological integration, which conscious attitudes often prevent'.[3]

Dream Interpretation

Jung believed, 'Dreaming has meaning, like everything else we do.'[4] He was a pioneer of dream interpretation: the decoding of dreams for comprehension by the rational mind.

Many of us try to decode our own dreams logically, but often we go about this in quite the wrong manner. The language of the dreaming mind is fundamentally irrational, so to attempt a logical translation of this alien tongue will yield poor results. The most important point from the perspective of analytical psychology is

---

* When we become lucid, the conscious mind is able not only to view the contents of the unconscious (as it does in non-lucid dreams) but also to interact with it face to face, in real time.

that 'when looking at a dream we should not forget that we are our dreams. We are the unconscious.'[5] Our rational mind needs to drop its expectations and linear logic if it wants to understand what the unconscious is offering. If we want to understand a dream ourselves, without the help of a trained analyst, we should 'try to immerse ourselves in the underlying energy, the feeling of the dream, so that it can slowly communicate itself and soak into our rational mind'.[6]

This process of basking in the atmosphere of a dream is a practice I call Dream Awareness. This is different from dream interpretation, because rather than trying to decode a meaning we allow the dream's essence to manifest spontaneously within our awareness. We will explore this practice further in Chapter 7.

TIBETAN BUDDHISTS ASLEEP

In Tibetan Buddhism, dreams are valued not as much for their content as for offering a potent training ground for spiritual practice – most importantly, an opportunity to recognize the illusion of the mind's projections. Rather than seeing them as a chance to process and integrate unconscious elements of the mind, Tibetan Buddhism focuses on the possibility of becoming enlightened as we sleep.

Buddhist scholar B. Alan Wallace says that within Buddhism it is believed that 'among the three general states of consciousness – waking, sleeping and dreaming – the coarsest state of consciousness, the one with the least potential for spiritual development is, surprisingly, the ordinary waking state'.[7] So, the dream and sleep states actually have more potential for spiritual development than daily life.

Tibetan Buddhism divides dreams into three main classes: ordinary samsaric dreams, dreams of clarity and clear light experiences.

Samsara is the term used to denote cyclic existence – the experience of birth, life, death and rebirth as perpetuated by dualistic ignorance. It is the antithesis of *nirvana*, enlightenment. Psychologically, it could be thought of as 'going round in circles', the repetition of fruitless emotional patterns and reactive mental narratives sourced from a belief in a permanently existing self. Samsaric dreams reflect this and simply consist of habits and memories from this life, and perhaps previous lives, too.

Dreams of clarity are decidedly different – they include what we in the West call lucid dreams and are considered very beneficial. They may range from witnessing dreams to high-level super-lucid dreams. They may also include dreams of significant insight (in which we may not necessarily be lucidly aware), prophetic dreams and the kind of transpersonal dream experiences that Carl Jung called 'big dreams'.

Clear light experiences go a significant step further. They are experiences in which we discover the true nature of our own mind, beyond, and apart from, our deluded projections, and beyond subject–object duality. To try to describe clear light experiences in words is a struggle, but it's safe to say that they are not so much dreams as experiences of non-dual awareness accessed through sleep.

To understand the Tibetan Buddhists' perspective on dreaming, it helps to understand what they mean by wakefulness. Wakeful experience is perceived not quite as the solid reality we persistently assume it to be, but rather as a dreamlike illusion, a subjective projection based on the impermanent, interdependent and contingent nature of all phenomena. It's not quite as simple as saying 'everything is a dream', more as if waking reality is viewed as dreamlike in nature and not as 'real' as we tend to regard it. Of course on a relative, everyday level things do exist – bills need to be paid and the laws of the universe apply – but on the level of enlightened understanding, waking life is not viewed as a fully awakened state but as a dreamlike mirage through which we are sleepwalking. In other words, in Tibetan Buddhism, the dream that we experience during sleep is actually a dream within a dream, or a 'secondary illusion' to the 'primary illusion' of waking life.

In his book *Sleeping, Dreaming, and Dying*, the Dalai Lama comments, 'If you ask why we dream, what's the benefit, there is no answer in Buddhism'[8] — other than its use in meditative practice.

So it could be said that from the perspective of Tibetan Buddhism, the benefits of dreaming are only truly met by engaging in meditative sleep practices such as lucid dreaming. Once we recognize that we are dreaming, the dream state can become a potential workshop of enlightened action and spiritual growth in which mindful awareness, compassionate action and the dissolution of negative mental tendencies can transform our very experience of existence.

We have now explored the question of why we dream from three different perspectives, and while the answers to why we dream may not be conclusive or comprehensive, the answers to why we would want to lucid dream are much clearer. The benefits alone should serve as sufficient inspiration to learn. Get ready to be inspired!

The Benefits of Lucid Dreaming and Mindfulness of Dream & Sleep

'There is no better way to show how our concept of reality can be blown away than through practising lucid dreaming.'
ROB NAIRN

As a child, on Sunday mornings I used to watch repeats of the old 1960s *Batman* series. I loved the dated fight scenes and I especially loved the Batphone – simply a pair of old-fashioned red telephones that gave Batman and Commissioner Gordon a secure line of communication. Whenever Commissioner Gordon needed Batman's help, he could call him directly. No engaged tones, no switchboards, no call waiting, no voicemail – just a clear line of two-way communication between the man who was seemingly in charge and the mysterious superhero.

Lucid dreaming is like having our own internal Batphone. Our conscious mind is like Commissioner Gordon (the man seemingly in charge) and our dreaming mind is like Batman (the mysterious superhero). Through lucid dreaming we can pick up our internal Batphone and communicate with the wellspring of wisdom that resides within our unconscious mind. This line of communication is direct, secure and never engaged, but always ready to help us better appreciate and understand ourselves. Each time we have a lucid dream we are strengthening this internal communication device so that with practice we are able to have conversations with wisdom so profound that it may well seem to reside outside us but in fact is at the very core of our being.

Through lucid dreaming we can communicate directly with seemingly tangible personifications of our own psychology. In the lucid dream state, our psychological concepts are often personified, or at least animated. This allows us to interact with them at a seemingly physical level. We can literally have a discussion with our higher self, meet our inner child or even offer a hug to the source of our deepest fear.

A LIBRARY OF KNOWLEDGE

Our dreaming mind holds within the unconscious a wealth of information about ourselves and the world around us. Rarely to be accessed in the waking state, this library of knowledge can be consciously accessed once we have a lucid dream. In a lucid dream we are literally walking around our own psyche, able to interact with aspects of our Self.

According to my friend the well-known hypnotherapy expert Valerie Austin, 'everything we have ever done, said, heard, smelled or seen is stored away in the subconscious'[1]* and hypnosis 'allows us access to this data straight from the subconscious without being edited by our rational conscious mind'.[2] A very similar process occurs during lucid dreaming.

It is not just through lucid dreaming and hypnosis that we can learn from our unconscious mind – it's trying to communicate

---

* Many people use 'subconscious' and 'unconscious' interchangeably, but I tend to use the term 'unconscious' when dealing with dreams, as this was the term that both Freud and Jung used.

with us every time we dream, lucidly or not. Lucid dreams are not in any way better than non-lucid dreams, they are just different. The library of knowledge that resides in our dreaming mind is open to us every time we dream and its content will be presented to us whether we are conscious of it or not. This is why it is good to practise dream awareness as well as lucid dreaming: by being more mindful of our dreams, we extend a hand of friendship to our deepest being. Dreaming is the most intimate relationship that we have with ourselves and every night our unconscious mind opens a window into our psyche through a narrative of symbols and imagery. In the words of Marc Barasch, author of *Healing Dreams*:

> *'Our dreams disturb us because they refuse to pander to our fondest notions of ourselves. Few forces in life present, with an equal sense of inevitability, the bare-knuckle facts of who we are, and the demands of what we might become.'*[3]

All too often these are communications that we either ignore or forget. But by learning how to appreciate and engage our dream world by simply bringing more mindfulness into our dreams and reflecting on them, let alone practising lucid dreaming, we begin to acknowledge a valid and valuable part of our life.

HEALING

I once met an ME sufferer who told me that she used lucid dreaming for healing. I instantly launched into an excited rant about how discoveries around neuropeptides* suggested that, at a cellular level, the mind did directly affect the body and how this opened up a huge vista of possibility for psychophysical

---

* Cellular biologist Bruce Lipton proposes in *The Biology of Belief* that neuropeptides (neuronal communicators located on cell membranes) directly affect the DNA within our cells, and that these neuropeptides are strongly influenced by our thoughts and feelings.

healing in the lucid dream state, infusing our very cells with healing energy…

'No, no, none of that!' she said.

She went on to describe how she used her lucid dreams to enjoy all the activities she couldn't do any more in the waking state. In her lucid dreams she went horse-riding, running and dancing, waltzing with her dreaming mind without the need for her wheelchair. This is but one example of the potential for psychological healing through lucid dreaming.

Often the healing is not just psychological. Many people believe in the potential for physical healing through visualization, such as the method in which patients imagine their body's immune system healing diseased cells in the form of coloured light.* Studies have shown that this kind of visualized healing can help to reduce stress, enhance the immune system and lessen pain[4] in many patients. These techniques are dependent upon our ability to visualize, something not all of us find so easy. In a lucid dream, however, the playing field is levelled, because a lucid dream is the most vivid and complete visualization we can experience. Applying those healing techniques within a lucid dream may prove far more effective than any visualization done in the waking state.

I've heard of lucid dreamers healing everything from warts on their feet to period pains and there is an overwhelming body of evidence in Robert Waggoner's book *Lucid Dreaming: Gateway to the Inner Self* to corroborate this. I myself have healed ear infections and torn ligaments through visualized healing in lucid dreams.** This will come as no surprise to dream yoga expert Dr Michael Katz, who says that while lucid, 'the power of the mind

---

* On his website, Dr David Hamilton cites a 2008 study published in the *Journal for the Society of Integrative Oncology* demonstrating how visualized healing can reduce the risk of recurrence of breast cancer.

** For a great example of physical healing through a lucid dream, see Dream 6, page 248.

is heightened', making visualized healing 'far more powerful than simply visualizing in the waking state'.[5]

There is also the potential to heal phobias within the lucid dream state using methods of gradual integration not dissimilar to those found in cognitive behavioural therapy. Phobias can be addressed by visualizing the source of the fear and then engaging with it in the knowledge that it is not real, just a mental projection. This new fearless engagement with the object of the phobia will leave a neurological pathway in the brain that may activate in the waking state, too, thus paving the way to curing the phobia for good.

As for addictions, these can be worked with in exactly the same way as you would in hypnotherapy. Just as a hypnotherapist might use the state of hypnosis as a way to contact the unconscious mind and offer it a beneficial suggestion pertaining to altering an addictive behaviour pattern, a lucid dreamer might use a lucid dream in a similar way. When we become lucid we are contacting the unconscious mind, as we are in hypnosis, but then moving even deeper still into its depths, meaning that if we call out, for example, *'I live a healthy lifestyle, I am a healthy, satisfied non-smoker now and forever more,'* in a lucid dream, this suggestion might work even more powerfully.

IMAGINARY REHEARSAL

My friend Rory MacSweeney had always dreamed of being a martial arts champion. In 1999 he made his dream come true by winning the gold medal at the European championships. When I say that Rory had always dreamed of being a champion, I'm not talking figuratively – he won his gold medal by training in his lucid dreams.

Although he kept up a rigorous daytime training regime for many years, he puts his winning edge down to the fact that while

41

his opponents were sleeping, in his lucid dreams he was sparring with dream characters and drilling advanced techniques that would create neurological pathways that could be engaged in the following day's training session.

In fact, any training while in the lucid dream state will create neural pathways that will carry over into the waking state, because our neurological system does not differentiate between lucid dream and waking experiences. This means that, just as we can use the 'total visualization' of the lucid dream state to heal, we can use it to train, too.

For decades sports scientists have been using waking-state imaginary rehearsal as a way to strengthen neural pathways. Only recently has the full potential of rehearsal within lucid dreams been explored. In 2005 a German research team at the University of Heidelberg was looking into lucid dream sports training with athletes and concluded that it led to improved performance in the waking state. The chief researcher of the project said the results far outperformed waking-state imaginary rehearsal and that 'training in a lucid dream can produce better results than visualized training in the waking state because in the lucid dream you experience your movements in a far more realistic way'.[6]

Other researchers agree and say that the main downside of waking visualization is that 'if the mental imagery technique is performed inadequately, without sufficient attention, subsequent gains in motor performance will be substandard'.[7] Lucid dreaming, however, solves this problem because it is the most complete visualization possible and allows for the most complete realization of the technique.

It's not just motor skills that can be honed through the strength of our imagination – we can actually strengthen our muscles, too.[8] Researchers at the Cleveland Clinic Foundation in 2004 asked a group of people to imagine lifting weights with their arms for

15 minutes a day, five days a week, for 12 weeks. At the end of their study, they concluded: 'Subjects who imagined lifting heavy weights with their arms increased their bicep strength by 13.5% on average and the gain in strength lasted for three months after they stopped the mental exercise regime.'[9]

If those gains in muscle strength were made through simple waking visualization, just imagine what gains could be made in the complete visualization of the lucid dream state. So, next time you're in a lucid dream, try doing a few press-ups – it might save you hours at the gym!

SELF-INCEPTION

In the Hollywood movie *Inception*, a group of special agents who can access people's dreams implant (or incept) suggestions in order to alter their waking consciousness and the decisions they make in their lives. Ideas are powerful and to self-incept an idea within our own dreaming mind can prove exceedingly effective.

When we become lucid we gain access to the fertile soil of the unconscious mind, so if we plant the seed of a beneficial idea or suggestion, it penetrates the deepest levels of our mind and affects our waking state in a tangible fashion. A lucid dream is the ideal environment in which to self-incept. In fact, within Tibetan Buddhism it is believed that 'the mind is up to seven times more powerful'[10] in the lucid dream state, so it's no surprise that self-inception works so well.

Whether it is by calling out beneficial statements of intent or engaging in new habit patterns such as generosity or fearlessness, new ideas and behaviour patterns can be implanted and implemented with full lucidity. For example, if you are painfully shy in waking life, you could go and interact with dream characters as a way to self-incept new habits of social confidence, or if you have a history exam the next day, an effective way to self-incept might be to call out, 'I am beneficially confident and assertive, with clear recall of any and all relevant facts pertaining to my history exam!'

Be creative, but be careful. I once self-incepted 'I am my full potential of health and fitness' within a lucid dream and woke up to insatiable cravings for raw fish, raw spinach and hard-core amounts of exercise which lasted for about six weeks after the dream. The unconscious will only give you what you are ready for, of course, but sometimes we underestimate just how ready for change we are!

WORKING WITH NIGHTMARES AND THE SHADOW
Nightmares

When I was 17 I had an accidental LSD overdose, which was terrifying and led to months of recurring post-traumatic stress nightmares. At the time I had just read one of my first lucid dreaming books and remembered the section on using lucidity to heal nightmares, but whenever I got lucid within these recurrent nightmares I was so consumed by fear and dread that I would usually just end up yelling, 'Wake up! I want to wake up!' Unfortunately this just happens to be the most effective way of ensuring that a nightmare recurs, because in no way does it resolve or heal the psychological trauma fuelling it.* At the time, however, I was simply too distressed to face my demons fearlessly.

One night I finally decided I'd had enough. I set a strong threefold motivation: to intentionally engage the nightmare, to become lucid within it and to face the source of the trauma.

That very night the nightmare came and the little bald-headed dwarf who had somehow come to represent the trauma appeared as usual, signifying imminent insanity. But this time I

---

* The most important thing to remember if you get lucid in a nightmare is this: *don't* try and wake yourself up. Stay in the dream for as long as you can and face the fear.

recognized that I was dreaming, and as he approached me, I finally turned to face him. Rather than run away, I yelled at him: 'Enough! I've had enough! OK, I get it! I see now! But please just leave me alone!'

Suddenly the dwarf's face changed and then the entire dreamscape changed into a 17-year-old's vision of paradise – in this case a beach full of bikini-clad girls and people skateboarding and drinking cocktails in the sun.

That was the last time I ever had that nightmare. Four months of post-traumatic stress cured by one lucid dream. It was then that I realized the huge potential of lucid dreaming.

For some people, chronic nightmares are a serious ailment that not only affects the quality of their sleep but also the quality of their lives. The good news is that if you can experience a nightmare with full lucidity, you have a powerful opportunity for trauma resolution and psychological integration, which is likely to lead to the cessation of the nightmares. In fact, at a meeting of the European Science Foundation in 2009 it was suggested that lucid dreaming was such an effective remedy for curing chronic nightmares that it could be offered as a mainstream treatment.[11] This means there may be a time in the future when doctors will give nightmare sufferers a prescription for lucid dream training rather than a prescription for medication.

Most people experience nightmares at some point in their lives, but usually it is not something they have to deal with all the time. Nevertheless, one thing that all of us do have to deal with constantly lies at the heart of our nightmares: the shadow.

The Shadow

The shadow is a Jungian concept used to describe the parts of the unconscious mind that are made up of all the undesirable aspects of our psyche that we have unconsciously rejected, disowned, repressed or denied. It is our dark side, comprised of everything within us that we don't want to face. Yet it is not evil or bad – it is merely the sum of those parts of us that are incompatible with who we think we are.*

We hide the psychological traits about ourselves from the world and from ourselves. We shove them into the recesses of our mind, where they gather, and from where they occasionally erupt, or spill forth when our guard is dropped. Preferring to remain unaware of our own shadow aspects, we find they become a dangerous influence, often lurking just beneath the surface. Jung said, 'Everyone carries a shadow, and the less it is embodied in the individual's conscious life, the blacker and denser it is.'[12]

However, although it contains our trauma, repressed sexuality and capacity for darkness, the shadow also represents a huge opportunity for the healing and acceptance practice known as shadow integration. Here we look into the darkness, acknowledging and accepting our own personal shadow aspects as a way to move towards psychological wholeness and balance. In Chapter 8, we will explore practically how we can use lucid dreaming for shadow integration, but fundamentally lucid dream shadow integration can be used to face our darkest fears and to deliberately engage nightmarish shadow aspects with compassionate acceptance rather than rejecting them. Shadow integration can be practised in the waking state, too, but it is much more direct when we do it in a lucid dream. For example, the memory of a childhood trauma that in the waking state might manifest as a heavy mental fog might appear in a lucid dream as a huge scary ogre. Whereas a mental fog can be difficult to pinpoint, and almost impossible to converse with, an ogre can be engaged with, questioned and even physically embraced.

---

* The shadow contains positive traits too. A young boy who has been caught dancing by his macho father and been chastised for it may well repress his inner dancer, and so his shadow might contain the very positive potential of creativity and dance.

This process of engaging shadow aspects with the aim of integrating and assimilating them into the self is part of what Jung termed individuation – the move towards psychological wholeness. This is one of the highest aims of psychological work, so we can see how lucid dreaming offers us an arena in which to reconnect with such deep levels of our psyche that when we wake in the morning, we may feel very different from the day before.

CREATIVITY

There is a great analogy in Richard Wiseman's book *59 Seconds* in which he describes our conscious and unconscious minds as being like two men sharing an office. One is loud, domineering and quite clever, but not very creative at all. He represents the conscious mind. The other is softly spoken but highly creative – representing the unconscious. If we were to ask them to come up with creative ideas on a certain subject, it's likely that the loud, uncreative one would bark out ideas, while the shy, creative genius wouldn't get a word in edgeways. The ideas might be quite good (the domineering man isn't an idiot), but they wouldn't be nearly as innovative as they would have been if the quiet, creative man had been allowed to contribute.

In waking life, when we are trying to make creative decisions, a similar scenario occurs, with our domineering conscious mind seldom allowing the creative genius of our unconscious mind to contribute. In dreams, however, we have a very different scenario indeed. The dream state is dominated by the unconscious mind. It is as if the loud guy has left the building while the quiet one has stayed on, working late, finally able to set his creativity free.

In terms of this metaphor, a lucid dream is like the loudmouth returning to the office a few hours later and finding that the shy genius has transformed their working environment into a whirlwind of creative activity. Suddenly his brash nature is subdued as he watches the quiet whizz-kid working masterfully. He finally appreciates how brilliantly creative his workmate is. He even decides he might ask his colleague's advice more often! If he does, he'll be likely to find him more than willing to offer help and ideas from the wellspring of his creative genius. This interaction might become the basis of an improved relationship between the two men.

If you want to tap into the infinite creativity of your unconscious, try becoming lucid so that your conscious mind can drop back into the office one night and listen to the advice of that shy but highly creative co-worker. (*For a great example of this co-worker in action, see Dream 13, page 256.*)

HAVING FUN!

Lucid dreaming allows you to do everything you've ever dreamed of doing. Whatever fantasy you choose, it's there for you in the hyper-realistic dream world of lucid awareness. You can be a movie star, have mad sexual orgies, experience psychedelic states and enjoy whatever your inner hedonist could wish for.

When I first taught myself to lucid dream at the age of 16, I used my newly found hobby for nothing more than sex, drugs and rock and roll. I wasted the first two years of my lucid dreaming practice almost exclusively on having sex in lucid dreams. At the time this felt like nothing more than harmless fun, and in fact it acted as a great motivational tool for me to get lucid as much as possible, but alas, it became a slippery slope down which I fell many times. For, as the great Irish poet W. B. Yeats said, 'In dreams begins responsibility.'[13] And in lucid dreams, even more so.

As in waking life, we are always creating and strengthening neural pathways while we are lucid dreaming, which means that if we engage in unbeneficial actions while lucid, we are creating neurological pathways associated with that action, which can then become activated in the waking state. Hence the slippery slope.

And if we consider the concept of karma (cause and effect), then once we're lucid, we have volition and conscious motivation – the two driving forces behind karmic imprints. This means karma is engaged in a similar way to when we are awake, so harmful acts in a lucid dream will leave negative karmic traces, just as they would in waking reality. So, have fun, but be careful what you get up to in the lucid dream state and try to treat it as a sacred space rather than a playground.

That said, it's not going too far to say that lucid dreaming is probably the most fun you can ever have. Flying, for example, feels as real as it would in the waking state. Like to travel? Try your hand at teleportation. Become invisible. Visit the moon. The sky is the limit. And remember, neuro-chemically, pleasure can be profoundly good for you, so if you've been running low on oxytocin, for example, maybe you've just been missing out on one of life's essential ingredients: fun!

It should now be easier to appreciate just how massive the potential of lucid dreaming is, for both physical and mental growth and wellbeing. So far we've concentrated mainly on the psychological benefits. But now let's move on to the spiritual benefits and see just how deep the rabbit hole goes.

PREPARATION FOR DEATH

Each day 150,000 people do it and one day we will do it, too. No matter where we're from or who we are, it is the one experience we will all share – the great equalizer. We will all do it and we will all do it successfully. We will all die. So, in the words of Dzogchen Ponlop Rinpoche,* we have a choice: 'to prepare ourselves to

---

* *Rinpoche* means 'precious one' in Tibetan and is used as a term of reverence for high lamas and esteemed masters. It is pronounced with an accent on the 'e' so that it rhymes with 'cabaret'.

face the most uncomfortable moment of our lives or to meet that moment unprepared'.[14]

Most of us in the West sleep for about 30 years of our lives, but how long do we spend contemplating death – an hour, a day, a week? I propose we start redressing this imbalance and start waking up to the reality of our mortality. While we are alive we have a wonderful opportunity to prepare ourselves for death and dying, so let's try and get over our defence mechanism of acting as though it's never going to happen and take some time to prepare.

One of the best preparations for death is through lucid dreaming and conscious sleeping. Within Tibetan Buddhism, as already mentioned, the main purpose of these sleep and dream practices is preparation for the dreamlike after-death *bardo* state. Each time we fall asleep and dream, we're getting a trial run for death and dying,* so every time we fall asleep consciously or have a lucid dream, we're training for the conscious recognition of the death process and the after-death *bardo*.

According to *The Tibetan Book of the Dead*, if we can manage to recognize the dreamlike hallucinations of the after-death *bardo* state as manifestations of the mind, we have the possibility of experiencing full spiritual awakening. It is said that even if a yogi has practised meditation for a whole lifetime and still hasn't attained full realization, he has one last shot at it: death.

My teacher and dream yoga master, Lama Yeshe Rinpoche, once told me, 'If you want to know how your mind will be during death, look at how your mind is during dream. If you can remember to recognize the dream consistently, then death means nothing to you, because you can recognize the death *bardo* as a dream, and then you can be with Buddha.' When it's

---

* Within the Tibetan teachings, the process of falling asleep corresponds to the dissolution of the four elements (earth, water, fire and air) which occurs at death.

4 a.m. and my alarm has gone off, reminding me to write down my dreams and practise lucid dreaming, it's that quote that spurs me on. Sure, we can use our lucid dreams to do loads of cool stuff that will help us while we're alive, but some of the greatest benefits of this practice come when we die.

SPIRITUAL PRACTICE

The great Tibetan masters also recommend that we use our lucid dreams to do spiritual practice such as meditation. In fact, doing spiritual practice in the lucid dream state is said to be so powerful that we have the potential to reach full enlightenment while we sleep. The first Karmapa, the spiritual head of the Karma Kagyu school of Tibetan Buddhism, attained full enlightenment at the age of 50 while practising dream yoga. So we shouldn't think that spiritual practice in the lucid dream state is somehow second best to waking practice – it can be even more effective. Dr Michael Katz testifies to this when he says that 'one moment of spiritual practice in a lucid dream is equivalent to one week of spiritual practice in the waking state'.[15]

What exactly is meant by 'spiritual practice' here? It's simple. Once lucid within a dream, engage in meditation, prayer, visualization, mantra recitation and so on in the same way that you would in the waking state. This is not only a great way to spend our dreaming hours, it's also incredibly powerful, because our dream body is unhindered by the physical limitations of our waking body, meaning that we have the potential to reach levels of accomplishment that may seem impossible in the waking state. Energy work such as *tai chi* or *chi gong* depends in part upon the movement and flow of energy through our body, which in the waking state can often be disrupted by internal blockages. In the lucid dream state, however, our dream body is pure energy with no physical form, which means that these types of energy practices can be engaged to their maximum potential.

In Tibetan Buddhism certain meditation practices require that we visualize ourselves taking on the actual form and qualities of a buddha, or an archetype of enlightened energy.

I've been doing these practices for years, and although my visualization has improved, I'm still not able to visualize myself in the form of a buddha with any real conviction in the waking state. However, if we engage in this within a lucid dream, we can transform into the actual form of the buddha and experience an aspect of that buddha's luminous nature. As soon as I became lucid one night, I visualized myself as the Buddhist archetype of compassion called Chenrezig, who is symbolized as a buddha with snow-white skin and four arms. Soon I started to feel an incredible buzzing sensation throughout my entire dream body. I felt as if I were exuding power from every pore, but a power of pure love and kindness. I then looked down at my dream body and was shocked to find that I now had snow-white skin and four arms! (*For a full description of this dream, see Dream 17, page 262.*)

Psychologically, this kind of practice leaves an indelible imprint on our mindstream, and physiologically, 'research shows that the dream environment is even more effective for establishing neural connections'[16] than waking visualization. So, our lucid dreams can reveal our limitless potential for enlightened manifestation. And, crucially, this serves to deepen our waking spiritual practice, too.

EXPLORING EMPTINESS

Shunyata, often translated as 'emptiness' or 'voidness', is a Buddhist term used to describe the impermanent and interdependent nature of all phenomena. What it suggests is that reality is in fact a dreamlike illusion, empty of all inherent solid existence.

I've heard some teachers say that *shunyata* should actually be translated as 'potentiality' – things are not empty because they are lacking something, but more because they contain infinite potentiality. Whichever way you look at it, the concept of *shunyata* is admittedly quite strange, even for practising Buddhists. As one Tibetan lama says, 'Emptiness will freak you out! Good freak out, but still freak you out!'[17]

It isn't just a concept, though – it has a practical application for our own happiness. Dzigar Kongtrul Rinpoche says that appreciating emptiness can help us to experience the world with a bit more flexibly because:

> **'When we understand that nothing exists independently, everything that does arise seems more dreamlike and less threatening. Because the nature of everything is emptiness, we can relax and enjoy the show.'[18]**

In a lucid dream we know that however solid, real and separate things may seem, they are actually an illusion created by our own mind. So, through lucid dreaming we directly experience a facet of emptiness. It is said that 'through dream yoga the yogi can directly recognize the emptiness of the personal self and of phenomena',[19] because if we can experience how convincingly real things are in our lucid dreams, we may become better able to experience the dreamlike nature of waking reality, too.

Through lucid dreaming we learn to combat grasping at the seemingly solid reality of waking existence, because we know what it feels like to be conscious within a similarly solid reality which we know is in fact an absolute figment of our imagination.

Seeing through the illusion of dualistic reality is all part of the process of spiritual awakening, but it is an experience that can be hard to muster in a world that seems so solid and separate from ourselves. A lucid dream offers us a rare training ground for this experience, because, as my teacher Rob Nairn once said, through lucid dreaming 'we experience the realization that what we thought to be real is actually not real, and so we are no longer experiencing the ignorance of the illusion. This is a taste of awakening.'[20]

If all this emptiness stuff seems a bit far out, it's worth noting that from the perspective of quantum physics, everything is empty. Well, 99.9999999999999 per cent empty, anyway. Only 0.00000000000001 per cent of an atom actually exists and the rest is empty space. Meaning that if we were to force together all the atoms of all the humans who had ever lived and then remove the empty space in those atoms, the entire human race would fit into an area the size of a sugar cube.[21] Now that really is far out.

RECEIVING TEACHINGS

Every one of us has an aspect of innate wisdom, often called the 'higher self' or 'enlightened potential', which is always within us. In the waking state, this inner wisdom can often seem quite hard to contact, but in a lucid dream it is much easier to access because the layers of ignorance that obscure our naturally enlightened mind are less dense.

While we are lucid, this inner wisdom will often offer us teachings spontaneously, taking on the form of an archetype of wisdom from our personal belief system – Jesus for one person, white light for another. Although the teachings may seem to come from a separate entity, they are, for the most part, sourced from within ourselves, from a potential that many of us are unaware we possess.

Having said that, we might also be able to receive teachings from the subtle energy mindstreams of enlightened beings. It seems to be far easier to tune into these mindstreams from the lucid dream state than from the waking state. Lama Tsongkhapa, the teacher of the first Dalai Lama, taught that one of the core aims of dream yoga was to receive teachings within the lucid dream from buddhas, enlightened masters and spiritual guides. Within this tradition, we are encouraged to request teachings from these enlightened sources once we are in a lucid dream.

In the Celtic tradition, seers spoke of 'thin places' – ley-line intersections or underground springs or other special sites where the boundary between the mundane and mystical was 'thin' and permeable. I believe that the lucid dream state is a similarly 'thin' place, with boundaries that are partially permeable, allowing us to access not only our own inner wisdom with greater ease but also the enlightened energy of other beings beyond those boundaries.

On many occasions I've called out for and received direct teachings within my lucid dreams from beings that appeared to be separate entities who had entered my dream state. Due to the interconnected nature of all things, of course these entities were as much projections of my own enlightened potential as they were seemingly separate from me.

But however they are delivered, are the teachings we receive in lucid dreams to be taken seriously? I believe that if they encourage us to be kinder and more compassionate to ourselves and others then we should put them into action – and only then. That's the safest option.

According to the great dream yogi Norbu Rinpoche, if we are truly aware in the dream state, a teaching received within the dream 'has the same value'[22] as a teaching received in the waking state, but he advises that we should apply discernment to all teachings, dream or waking, rather than accepting them out of blind faith.

MINDFULNESS TRAINING

Mindfulness is one of the fastest-growing forms of meditation practice in the West and has been scientifically proven to improve health, happiness and overall wellbeing. We'll explore mindfulness meditation in Part II, but for now it is enough to say that mindfulness is all about awareness. By training ourselves to be more aware, we naturally become kinder and happier, because almost all of our unkindness, to ourselves and others, stems from a lack of mindful awareness. It is said that 'in a state of mindfulness, you see yourself exactly as you are. You pierce right through the layer of lies that you normally tell yourself and you see what is really there.'[23]

Training ourselves to be more mindful is one of the greatest gifts we can give ourselves and others, but we don't just learn this by sitting down to meditate. Through lucid dreaming and conscious sleeping we can train ourselves to develop our capacity for mindful awareness while we sleep.

The essence of mindfulness meditation is 'knowing what is happening while it is happening, without judgement',[24] so lucid dreaming is not just analogous to mindfulness meditation but is actually a direct extension of it. Lucid dreaming requires a constantly vigilant mindful awareness that has to be maintained throughout the dream, which is exactly what is required in waking mindfulness practice.

Daytime meditation practice was the original lucid dream induction technique, and it has long been known that mindfulness during waking leads to mindfulness during dreaming. What is less known is that it works the other way around, too.

Dr Akong Rinpoche, the man who co-founded Samye Ling, the first Tibetan Buddhist centre in the West, told me how this process worked. Usually a man of few words, he described in detail how these practices actually helped to strengthen waking mindfulness: 'People in the west don't know that sleep is a place in which to train the mind. Dream yoga is all about mind training. It is about how not to lose your mind during sleep, and is instead used to train the mind to maintain its all-round capacity for mindful awareness.'[25]

LUCID LIVING

I have a friend named Timothy Freke. He often says, 'With a name like mine, I guess I had to become a philosopher.' And so he did. Tim's areas of expertise focus mainly on Christian Gnosticism and the concept of lucid living that the Christian Gnostics proposed. Waking up to life and living lucidly was a central concept for these mystic proto-Christians, as we can see from their call to 'Wake up! Rouse yourself from the collective coma that you mistake for "real life"!'[26]

The Gnostics believed that we were sleepwalking through the illusion of waking reality, unaware that it was all just as empty of inherent existence as our dreams. If only we could wake up in this life and get lucid in our waking reality, maybe then we would see that life was but a dream? When I talk about lucid living and waking up to life, I'm talking about awakening in the same way that the Buddha did. As Buddhist scholar Stephen Batchelor says, the Buddha wasn't talking about waking up to some sort of absolute reality or God as such, but rather about waking up 'to the unfolding of the phenomenal world itself… awakening to the flux and the flow, the pain, the beauty, the tragedy and the joy of life itself'.[27]

Far from trying to wake up, most of us actually willingly surrender 30 years of our life to non-awareness. Each night we fall into an abyss of ignorance, surrendering six to eight hours to unconsciousness, and then wake up in the morning as if this is the most natural thing in the world. We are in fact conditioned to see it as normal and to view sleep as a time of complete non-awareness, a time to 'switch off the computer', but it doesn't have to be this way.* Although much of sleep *is* about the body and brain shutting down, the time spent in dreaming sleep is not, and so, as the dream yogi Tenzin Rinpoche says, 'These dream

---

* Much of sleep is about restoration, but we don't have to be unconscious for this restoration to occur. Conscious sleeping and lucid dreaming practices will make our sleep more refreshing, not less so.

practices can help us not to waste that time but to spend it learning to discover our inner potential. What a fantastic tool!'[28]

When I teach people that they may be losing 30 years to total lack of awareness, they often reply, 'Yeah, maybe, but at least I'm wide awake and living lucidly for the rest of it!' Unfortunately this simply isn't true. New studies from a Harvard University research team have found that most people are unaware and not in the present moment for 47 per cent of their waking lives.[29] The researchers concluded that most of us live our lives on autopilot, lost in fantasy and very rarely present and mindful. Most of us are definitely not living lucidly, but every time we have a lucid dream we are habituating the mind to be more aware and more lucid than usual.

In a lucid dream of course we become aware that what we believed to be real (the dream) is not real but just a mental projection. By becoming lucid, we see through our projections, and each time we do that we are creating a habitual tendency towards seeing through our projections in the waking state, too.

In the Freudian sense, 'projection' describes a psychological defence mechanism in which we unconsciously project our own unacceptable qualities onto others. For example, if we are arrogant, we may deny this in ourselves but see it in others to a degree not quite proportionate to reality. The arrogance of others becomes exaggerated in our eyes and this 'pushes our buttons'. In fact, what annoys us most in other people is often a trait we are working hard not to recognize and accept in ourselves. Once we establish a stabilized lucid dreaming practice, however, we are engraining a new power of recognition that can 'see through' projections, not only of the dream type but of the waking type, too.* This is how we begin to live lucidly, because

---

* The first time I experienced this it was just like becoming lucid in a dream. I had a sudden flash of awareness as I became conscious of projecting my own insecurity onto someone as I was talking to them.

we start to recognize our waking psychological projections in the same way as we recognize our dreams.

Through learning to dream lucidly, we can learn to live lucidly and wake up to life. Perhaps we can even realize what those early Gnostic Christians were getting at when they said, 'Wake up. How can you bear to be asleep when it's your responsibility to be awake?'[30]

PART II
PATH

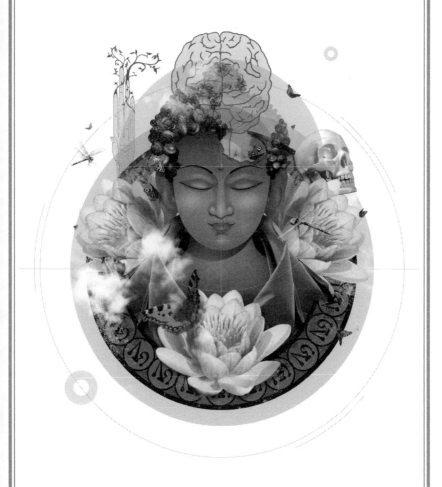

Lucid Dreaming Techniques

'We're dreaming?'
*'You're actually in the middle of the workshop
right now, sleeping. This is your first lesson...
Stay calm.'*
<small>INCEPTION</small>

Now that we've prepared the ground, answered some of the most frequently asked questions and have a broad outline of the history and benefits of the practice, it's time to move on to the actual path of lucid dreaming and Mindfulness of Dream & Sleep. This part of the book aims to leave you with a toolbox of techniques with which you can learn to dream lucidly. We'll look at everything from how to engage in conscious sleeping, to what to do once you get lucid, how to maintain your lucidity and how to use obstacles as opportunities.

The practices that we will explore here are taken from both Western and Tibetan Buddhist sources. Although many Tibetan dream yoga techniques can't be shared outside a formal retreat setting, don't feel that you're missing out on the complete package, because, as one high lama says, 'Training in dream yoga is similar to the methods developed by Western researchers. Both the Western exercises and the Tibetan methods can be used, since they are essentially the same thing.'[1]

I've seen the following practices transform people's lives and help to bring into their waking state a lucid awareness that radiates humour and warmth in all directions.

The lucid dreaming training methods in this chapter are some of the well-known Western and LaBergian techniques, plus a few new ones of my own. Established lucid dreamers will be well aware of many of these techniques already, but I have added to and expanded upon them somewhat, mainly by placing them into a context of mindfulness training.

These techniques can be practised by people of all faiths and levels of ability, and each one has been tested, refined and successfully applied by the thousands of dreamers around the world I've taught at retreats, workshops and lectures.

To learn any new skill, the brain requires consistent repetition of the new action in order to strengthen and eventually hardwire the neural pathways associated with that new action. So, effort, motivation and intention are the bedrock of a stable lucid dreaming practice. It's not about faith, it's about determination.

Charlie says

'Getting lucid won't happen just by reading about lucid dreaming – it's all about practising lucid dreaming. Just as looking at a map won't get you anywhere, reading this book won't give you lucid dreams – you need to set out on the path.'

WHAT'S YOUR MOTIVATION?

Stephen LaBerge famously said that there were three essential requirements for learning to lucid dream: excellent *dream recall,* correct practice of *effective techniques* and *strong motivation.* The dream recall and effective techniques can be taught, but the motivation is down to each one of us individually.

So, is your motivation just to have a bit of fun or to try to make use of your sleep for psychological growth? Either option is fine, but there's a third option, too: to use these practices to wake up to your highest potential.

The Tibetan Buddhist masters say that we should try to imbue our dream practice with 'bodhicitta* motivation', which means that we are motivated to have lucid dreams not just for our own benefit but to awaken our deeper capacity for wisdom and compassion, which will benefit other beings, too. That seems a pretty sensible motivation, whether you're a Buddhist or not, but how can lucid dreaming be used to benefit others? It's said that every time you become lucid, wisdom is accumulated, because you are gaining insight into illusion and training your capacity for mindful awareness, which is the bedrock for love and compassion. Essentially, by becoming lucid in our dreams, we become more lucid, insightful and compassionate in our waking life – and that can only benefit others.

Charlie says

'Lucid dreaming makes us kinder in everyday life. It shows us how our mind creates illusion, which allows us to see how other people's minds do the same. Once we see that, we realize that everybody is trying their best and that we're all in this together. We become a bit more tolerant and responsive, rather than closed and reactive.'

* Bodhicitta is one of the most important aspects of Tibetan Buddhism. It's the wish to attain enlightenment not just for oneself, but for the benefit of all beings (Sanskrit: *bodhi* = enlightened essence; *citta* = heart/mind).

DREAM RECALL

It took me years to appreciate fully just how vital dream recall is to lucidity. Initially, I thought it was just a way of making sure you remembered your dreams and a stepping stone to more advanced techniques. This isn't the case, though. Training in dream recall is essential, whatever your position on the path.

Why don't most people remember their dreams? There are all sorts of theories on this, ranging from it being maladaptive for early humans to remember their dreams (in case they confused them with reality) to ineffective modern sleeping patterns to a disregard for dreams in general, but I believe the reason people don't normally remember their dreams is simply because they don't try to remember them.

Charlie says

'Everybody dreams every night, but not everybody remembers their dreams. If you don't remember your dreams, that's probably because you've never tried to remember them! When did you last think I really want to remember my dreams?'

Dream recall is like ploughing the field of our unconscious, preparing it for the seeds of the lucidity techniques. We could just chuck a few seeds onto the field – a few might sprout – but if we plough the field properly we'll get a much bigger harvest.

Dream recall is a great memory practice, too. It trains the mind to remember what it was up to while we were asleep and because it encourages us to flex our mindful memory muscles as soon as we wake up, it's great for our all-round mental health.

If we set a strong intention to recall our dreams, most of us will be able to recall them without too much difficulty after just a couple of nights. It's all about intent.

Here are a few ways to boost your recall:

- Knowing the time of your REM periods can be a great way to increase your recall, because if you wake people from REM sleep, about 95 per cent of them will be dreaming and will be able to describe what they were dreaming about.[2] So, if you want to remember your dreams, try waking yourself during a REM period. REM periods get longer and occur at shorter intervals as the night progresses, so set an alarm clock for some time during the last two hours of your sleep cycle to have the best chance of waking up with dream recall. (*For more information, see 'The Stages of Sleep', page 95.*)

- Many people try and recall their dreams after the dream has happened. This often doesn't work very well. It's much better to set your intention to recall your dreams *before* you start dreaming. As you fall asleep, set a strong intention to remember your dreams and fall asleep reciting the suggestion 'Tonight, I remember my dreams. Tonight I have excellent dream recall.' This simple method can be a profoundly effective remedy for dream amnesia.

- Dream memories often seem to be stored in the muscle memory of our physical body, so for optimal dream recall, don't move from the position in which you wake up until you can recall the dream. If you do have to move your body, to press the alarm clock for example, return to the position in which you woke up and focus on recalling your dream from there.

- Dream yogis say, 'Like a ball of yarn, even if we can only get the very end of the thread, we can work backwards and eventually unravel the entire dream.' So, even if you can only recall one fact or theme of the dream, you can work backwards from that point, eventually gathering the rest of the dream. As soon as you wake up, ask yourself: 'Where was I? What was I just doing? What was I dreaming about?'

- You can improve your dream recall by improving your waking recall, so train your memory muscles by memorizing your 'to do' list or remembering phone numbers off by heart or even playing brain-training video games.

Some people remember their dreams naturally, but for others it may take several days or even weeks of mental effort to do so. Whatever the state of your current dream recall, work with what you have and progress from there. Even if you can only recall a few fragments from each dream, that's a great start.

KEEPING A DREAM DIARY

Keeping a dream diary is as simple as this: whenever you wake up from a dream, recall as much of the dream as you can and then write it down. You don't need to document every tiny detail; you'll know what feels worth noting and what doesn't. Focus on the main themes and feelings, the general narrative and any strange dream anomalies that you can recall. If you were recalling dreams for dream interpretation then you might want to document the dream in more detail, but you aren't, you're recalling them so that you get to know the territory of your dreams, the feel of your dreams and the shape of your dreams – three aspects that will help you to recognize your dreams lucidly.

Nowadays many people type their dreams onto their tablet or phone, but for others nothing beats a good old pen and paper. If you're going to write up your dreams by hand, buy a notebook with paper that is a pleasure to write on, and use a pen that writes easily – do everything you can to encourage yourself to use it regularly.

Be sure to record the date of each dream at the top of the page* and feel free to give each dream a title – one that encapsulates it.

---

* The importance of the date is so that once you start to have lucid dreams you can chart your progress, and even cross-refer your dream diary with your everyday diary to see how your daily life influences your dreams.

The Benefits of Keeping a Dream Diary

- It comes down to this: 'the more conscious you are of your dreams, the easier it will be to become conscious within your dreams'.[3]

- Writing down your dreams pays homage to the dreams and, more importantly, reinforces the habit of viewing dreams as something valuable. Once you see dreams as valuable you will naturally start to recall them with more ease and your dreaming mind may even respond by giving you dreams of more psychological value.

- Through the act of actually writing down your dreams you are recognizing the memory of an unconscious process with your conscious awareness. So your dreams will manifest in a more conscious and recognizable way. *Recognizable* is the key word here, because the point of all these practices is to recognize that you are dreaming while you are dreaming.

- By recalling your dreams, you're getting to know the territory of your dreaming mind. The better you get to know that territory, the more likely you are to recognize it when you're in it and become lucid.

Top Tips for Dream Diaries

- Write down your dreams as soon as you remember them. Don't wait until the morning – do it straightaway. Countless times I've heard people say that they woke up in the night and recalled their dream so strongly that they were sure that they would still remember it in the morning, but in the morning it was gone!

- It can seem pretty hectic to scrabble around for your dream diary at 5 a.m., but you'll soon find the least disruptive method for you. Whether it's going to the bathroom to write up your dreams or having a little torch by your bedside to avoid waking your partner, you'll find a way. Many people avoid having to switch the light on at all by typing their dreams into their mobile phone and then printing them out at the end of each month.*

- Whether you can afford half an hour documenting your dreams each morning or only five or ten minutes, either option is fine but make sure you stick to it.

- Mind maps, illustrations, spider diagrams and artwork can all be incorporated into your dream diary. The important thing is to recall the dream, not so much how it is recalled.

- Voice recorders should be avoided if possible, though, because although it's difficult to 'sleep write', we can 'sleep talk'. If you try to record your dream into a voice recorder and you're not fully awake, you may well end up with a recording of yourself falling asleep!**

Charlie says

'Apart from leading to lucid dreams, keeping a dream journal gives you a nightly insight into the state of your mind. If you really want to know your own psychology, look at your dreams. They're an uncensored snapshot of you at that moment of your life. A dream journal is far more honest than a daytime journal, because your dreams don't lie.'

Before you get into the next set of practices, make sure that your dream recall is quite solid. Without regular dream recall you might find some of the following techniques hard to engage in. You can still give them a shot, but without good dream recall that might be a shot in the dark.

---

* If you choose this method, be sure you back up the files or use an online cloud storage system.

** In his book *59 Seconds*, Professor Richard Wiseman says, 'Talking can often be more unstructured, disorganized and by its nature improvised, in contrast to writing, which is more systematic and organized around structure.'[4]

DREAM SIGNS

Once we've begun to recall our dreams, we can move on to spotting dream signs. A dream sign is any improbable, impossible or bizarre aspect of dream experience that can indicate that we're dreaming. Often our dreams are full of dream signs, which can range from as subtle as being back in our childhood school to as obvious as flying pink elephants. If it's something that doesn't usually occur in waking life, then it's a potential dream sign.

There are hundreds of different types of dream sign, but I classify them into three main groups:

- anomalous: random one-off anomalies such as walking trees or barking cats;

- thematic: dreamlike themes or scenarios such as being back at school or being naked in public, rather than specific objects or characters;

- recurring: dream signs that have appeared in two dreams or more.

By keeping a dream diary, we can recognize and record our particular dream signs and make notes of any recurring ones. Acknowledging our particular dream signs in the waking state will lead to the conscious recognition of them within the dream state, thus triggering lucidity.

Let's Spot Dream Signs!

Once you've recalled and documented a dream, read back through it, looking for any dream signs. If you read 'I was in a café on the moon with my dead grandmother being served tea by a talking dog', your dream signs will be 'café on the moon', 'dead grandmother' and 'talking dog'. If this is the second or third time that you've dreamed about your dead grandmother, then 'dead grandmother' will be a recurring dream sign.

Once you've pinpointed your dream signs, make a determined effort to be on the lookout for any future anomalies that might indicate that you're dreaming. This determined effort will seep into your dreams and eventually you'll start recognizing dream signs from within the dream.

If you spot a recurring dream sign, firmly resolve to use it as a *lucidity trigger* by saying to yourself before bed: 'The next time I see my dead grandmother, I'll recognize that I'm dreaming and become lucid.' Then of course, when you next dream about your dead grandmother, the lucidity trigger will be activated, making you spontaneously think *Am I dreaming? Aha! This is a dream sign, I must be dreaming!* and you will become lucidly aware.

One of the most common entries into a lucid dream is simply to spot a dream sign and become lucid. But sometimes, even though you've spotted a dream sign and are sure that you must be dreaming, the rest of the dream will look so realistic that you simply can't accept that you're in a dream. This is when you need reality checks.

REALITY CHECKS

'You must start by doing something very simple. Tonight in your dreams you must look at your hands.'

Don Juan, Yaqui Indian dream master[5]

This is where it all gets a bit strange. The Lucidity Institute has scientifically verified that there are certain things that are virtually impossible for the human mind to consistently replicate *within* the pre-lucid dream state* and so these can be used to reliably confirm whether or not you're dreaming. There are loads of them, but here are some of my favourites:

---

* Reality checks will almost always be performed in the pre-lucid dream state, because if you are conscious enough to think *I should do a reality check*, then you are often already pre-lucid.

- Looking at your outstretched hand twice in quick succession without it changing in some way;

- Reading text coherently twice without it changing in some way;

- Using digital or electrical devices without them changing or malfunctioning in some way.

When I first read about these reality checks I thought they were a load of hokum (perhaps as you do now?), but try and stay with me on this because once you know how they work it all makes sense.

During a dream, the brain is working flat out to maintain the projection of our elaborately detailed dreamscape in real time, and although it's amazingly good at this, once pre-lucid it struggles to replicate the detailed minutiae of an intricate image (such as a piece of text or an outstretched hand) twice in quick succession. So, if we try and make it engage in such a replication, it will provide a close but imperfect rendering, and it's the acknowledgement of this imperfect rendering that makes us lucidly aware.

Let's Check Reality!

Looking at your hands: if you think you might be dreaming, look at your outstretched hand within the dream, then quickly look away and look back at it again.* Alternatively, watch your hand as you flip it over and back again. Either way, your brain will struggle to reproduce an identical projection of your hand, so upon second glance it may be a strange shape, perhaps missing a finger or two, or look dappled or transformed. The dreaming brain tries its best to reproduce exactly the same image, but doesn't quite have the

---

* This is one of the most applicable reality checks because most people are embodied in their dreams and so a hand is always within reach. Of course there are loads of other reality checks, so feel free to improvise.

processing speed to do so perfectly. The variations are multiple, but the result is singular: if you really expect your hand to change, it will change.*

Reading text: within a pre-lucid dream it is virtually impossible to read any text coherently twice in succession. LaBerge's research laboratory found that in lucid dreams text changed 75 per cent of the time as the dreamer was reading it and 95 per cent of the time on second reading.[7] So, if you think you might be dreaming, try to read something. The text will often be unintelligible, move around as you're reading it or in some cases just fade away altogether. All these are signs that you're dreaming.**

Using digital and electrical appliances: just as the mind struggles to reproduce text, so it also struggles with the highly detailed screen of a mobile phone or computer, which will often seem blurred and fluid in a pre-lucid dream as the dreaming mind struggles to project it accurately. Similarly, it is virtually impossible to read a digital watch, successfully operate any form of digital or electrical appliance or switch a light on and off. This works on the principle that if you flick a light switch within a dream you're asking the dreaming mind to project an exact replication of the dreamscape but in a totally different light and shadow setting, literally at the flick of a switch. This is something that it finds almost impossible to do.

---

* When Castaneda presses his teacher Don Juan about why he should look at his hands in particular, Don Juan replies, 'You can of course look at whatever you goddam please – your toes, your belly or even your pecker!'[6] I would still recommend your hands though.

** Perhaps this can be explained in part by the well-documented phenomenon whereby people recognize most words by their shape and so it *deosn't mttaer waht oredr ltteers appaer, olny taht the frist and lsat ltteers are in the rghit pclae.*

> **Charlie says**
>
> *'You're in a dream and you think you might be dreaming. You look at your hand, flip it over with the expectation that it will change if you are dreaming, and when you flip it back, it probably will have changed. I've had my hand turn into a tree, a robotic claw, a balloon and even just a stump of flesh. The dreaming mind is very creative, but it's not very good at replicating precise detail. Hands are pretty detailed, so it really struggles to replicate them to order.'*

The Neuroscience behind Reality Checks

Until you've actually experienced doing a reality check, it can seem quite far-fetched, but let neuroscience put your mind at ease. Dreaming is mainly a right-brain activity; the logical left brain is almost entirely offline while we dream. But when it comes to detailed information-processing, such as fluent reading, recognition of complex symbols and identifying detailed patterns, we rely almost solely on the superior processing speed of our left brain.[8] So the left brain contains the program for 'how to read' and 'how to recreate detailed patterns', but because it is almost entirely offline while we dream, if we try to process detailed patterns, we'll be stumped. Working on this basis, we can see why all the reality checks that involve fluent reading and recreating detailed patterns are especially difficult within the dream state.

This book contains quite a few techniques that engage the respective specialities of the left and right hemispheres of the brain, so before we move on it's worth having a look at these hemispheres more closely. A few years back we could get away with saying that the left brain *only* does this and the right brain *only* does that, but advancements in brain imaging technology now show that it's not that clear cut. However, we can definitely still say that the left hemisphere deals *more* with logical, calculating tasks, whereas the right hemisphere deals *more* with imaginative, creative tasks. It's as if your headspace is shared by both an artist and an accountant. The left hemisphere also contains the 'I am' program, the basis of our egocentric sense of self, whereas the right hemisphere contains a potential for interconnected oneness that is usually subjugated by the dominance of the left brain and its 'I am' motherboard. Neuroscientist Jill Bolte Taylor says that the right hemisphere operates like a parallel processor (it can carry out multiple tasks simultaneously), but the left is like a serial processor (it carries out individual tasks in sequence), and although the two hemispheres do communicate through the *corpus callosum*, the link between the two, they are in many ways each quite unique.

Interestingly, research has shown that once we actually have the 'Aha!' moment of lucidity, left-hemisphere brain function comes back online within about 30 seconds,[9] meaning that reality checks may become less noticeable as the lucid dream progresses.

Charlie says

'Don't get too hung up on all this left/right-brain stuff. All you need to know is that hands, text, detailed patterns and electrical gizmos do weird things in the dream state. If you can recognize that weirdness as it happens then you'll know that you're dreaming. You don't need a neuroscientist to tell you that.'

Although opportunities for reality checks will often crop up in your dreams naturally, they are usually only engaged once you spot a dream sign and need confirmation of your present reality. You can, however, actively hasten the process by getting into the habit of conducting reality checks while you're awake. This habit will naturally carry over into your dreams, so that soon you will actually *dream* about doing a reality check. This is the basis of the Weird technique…

THE WEIRD TECHNIQUE

This technique is deceptively simple, but it's how I have the majority of my lucid dreams. From now on, in the daytime, whenever something weird happens or whenever you experience synchronicity, *déjà vu*, a strange coincidence or any other type of dreamlike anomaly, ask yourself, 'Am I dreaming?' and then answer this question by doing a reality check.

By doing reality checks during the daytime, while you're awake, you're creating a habit that will then reappear in your dreams. But when you dream about doing a reality check, it will of course indicate that you're dreaming and lead to lucidity.

Fascinatingly, lucid dreaming specialist Daniel Love has calculated that '11% of our mental experience each day is spent dreaming'.[10] He goes on to say, 'Just to clarify, this is not 11% of sleeping activity but 11% of your entire daily experience each and every day.'[11] This means that every time we apply the Weird technique we have about a one in ten chance that we will actually be dreaming. I like those odds.

• •

Let's Look for Weirdness! 🦋🦋

In the waking state, whenever something strange or unusual happens, ask yourself, 'Am I dreaming?' and then answer the question by doing a reality check such as looking at your hand twice in quick succession or reading a piece of text twice in a row. If you do this ten or more times a day, it seems to be enough for you to start dreaming about doing it and so lead you to lucidity.

'As we live, so we dream', so don't just flip your hand over flippantly every time something odd happens, because that's what will happen in your dreams too, rendering the technique useless. Be sure to act with full conviction and the expectation that the reality check will come back positive if you are actually dreaming.

Charlie says

'A woman on one of my courses once said, "You want me to go around all day asking, 'Am I dreaming?' and looking at my hands to check if I'm awake? That'll send us all mad!" It's actually quite the opposite though – every time we do a reality check we're practising mindfulness because we're taking a moment to stop, come into the present moment and become more aware of our current reality. Every time we acknowledge something strange happening in the waking state and do a reality check, we're coming back into the present moment and coming out of autopilot mode.'

Pre-lucid Confabulation

Sometimes as beginners we might find ourselves in a dream, spotting a dream sign, about to become lucid… and then talk ourselves out of it. Other times we think we might be dreaming and do a reality check but then become distracted by the dream before we can become lucid. This bizarre phenomenon is what I call 'pre-lucid confabulation'.

I was talking about confabulation at a retreat in Wales once when a psychologist from the audience said under her breath, 'Bullshit!'

I stopped, looked at her and said, 'Excuse me?'

She replied, 'Bullshit! Confabulation is all about bullshit. We bullshit ourselves in order to maintain the status quo of our reality. Psychotics do it all the time.'

It seems that when we are confronted by the possibility of recognizing that we're dreaming, our egoic sense of self often tries to confabulate a seemingly rational explanation for the reality of the situation. For example, we might see a flying elephant and be on the cusp of lucidity, but then convince ourselves that flying elephants are quite common in this part of the world.

Why would our egoic sense of self do this? Because it feels threatened by lucidity. Once we're lucid, we see through the illusion of our egoic sense of self and become part of the dream, beyond any notions of me, my, I and 'other'. We are in fact one with everything in the dream and so the stranglehold of the egoic self is released. To prevent this, out of misjudged desperation it sometimes tries to stop us from becoming lucid.

In the Castaneda text *The Art of Dreaming*, the protagonist Don Juan tells his student that our rational mind will try to protect itself if we encounter ideas or concepts in our dreams that seek to usurp our notion of accepted rationality. This idea of rationality fighting for its own survival in the face of irrational dream experiences is one that beginner lucid dreamers may sporadically encounter, often in the form of dream characters denying that they are 'the stuff of dreams' as our rational mind tries to maintain control over the dreaming status quo.

Luckily, as our lucid dreaming practice progresses and our use of reality checks increases, the frequency of confabulation decreases, but beginners, beware – once you suspect that you might be dreaming, don't accept any facts to the contrary without checking them thoroughly. Just like Lieutenant Columbo.

THE COLUMBO METHOD

No reality-check technique works 100 per cent of the time, so what do you do if your hand doesn't change but you're still sure you're dreaming? How can you do the reading reality check if there isn't any text to read in the dream? How can you spot a dream sign if the dreamscape is seemingly devoid of them?

Sometimes you might find yourself in a scenario where both recognition of dream signs and reality checks seem null and void and yet you still have a gut feeling that you might be dreaming. This is when you need to rely on checking the facts and looking closely at your surroundings, like a detective scanning a crime scene. This is the basis for the Columbo Method.

For those of you old enough to remember him, think back to the 1970s TV detective Lieutenant Columbo. He was a cigar-smoking LAPD detective who represented every man (and woman)'s bumbling inner detective. Columbo didn't have flashy forensics or complicated theories, he just used his own sound judgement and awareness to detect the reality of a situation.

Columbo could walk into a room and notice ten clues before he'd even introduced himself; he had a broad awareness that took in every detail of the environment while remaining totally relaxed, not giving anything away, innocently puffing on his Cuban cigar. That's just how we need to be if we want to solve the mystery of the lucid dream.

Let's Search for Clues! 🦋

Once you suspect that you might be dreaming, look for evidence of dreaming just like a detective searching an area for clues. Be mindful, be aware, be vigilant. Try asking yourself, 'How did I get here? Where was I before I arrived here?' and 'look for rifts in cause and effect... and any impossibilities',[12] which will help you detect the dream state.

While you are searching for these clues, try to stay totally cool and calm, just like Columbo, because if you get overexcited you may either wake up or give the game away, leading to the possibility of confabulatory new dream material that will uphold the illusion of the dream.

To really empower the Columbo Method, practise it in the daytime, too. As you go through your daily life, or perhaps for a designated 10 minutes a day, look very closely at things, feel the textures around you, investigate odd-looking places and examine your experience in depth. You can even ask yourself, 'How did I get here?' at regular intervals throughout the day. If you do these types of engaged mindfulness practice often enough, you'll end up doing them in your dreams, too.

Charlie says

'If you think you might be dreaming, look closely! Scan the area for clues, touch things, engage the space, be mindful. The dream state looks amazingly realistic, but if you look closely enough you'll be able to see the dreamlike inconsistencies and recognize that you're dreaming.'

LABERGE'S MILD (MNEMONIC INITIATED LUCID DREAM) TECHNIQUE

Mnemonic means 'pertaining to memory' and a Mnemonic Initiated Lucid Dream is one that works by using the function of memory. MILD was the technique Stephen LaBerge developed that allowed him to have lucid dreams at will. Many people find it one of the most effective lucid dreaming technique there is.

The MILD technique is based upon the principles of visualization, autosuggestion (self-hypnosis) and prospective memory. Interestingly, the basis of the technique can be found in a 16th-century dream yoga text by Lochen Dharma Shri,[13] but a full explanation of the modern version can be found in *Exploring the World of Lucid Dreaming* by Stephen LaBerge.

Although visualization and autosuggestion provide the foundational power of this technique, it is prospective memory that provides the real crux. We use prospective memory all the time in daily life when we say things like 'Next time I see a bank I'll remember to get out some cash.' And it's actually a very reliable aspect of memory.* If we use it with strong intent, we activate the motivational or goal-seeking part of the brain, which will stay unconsciously activated throughout both waking and sleep states until that goal is achieved. In the same way, a prospective memory command that we set as we fall asleep, such as 'Next time I'm dreaming I'll remember to recognize that I'm dreaming' will stay neurologically engaged until we next find ourselves dreaming.

MILD is a technique that requires us to visualize ourselves back in the dream that we were just having and so is best practised after waking from a vividly recalled dream. This can be done naturally, perhaps when you've woken up in the early hours, or intentionally, by setting an alarm to wake yourself up during a REM period sometime in the last few hours of your sleep cycle.**

Let's Get MILD! 🦋🦋

1. Recalling the dream: after awakening from a period of dreaming, wake up fully and recall the dream that you were just having. Learn the basic plot and scenario off by heart and then if possible choose a scene or part of the dream that has a dream sign in it. Memorize this part of the dream. You'll find out why in step 3.

2. Setting the intent: now get ready to go back to sleep. As you begin to fall asleep and enter the hypnagogic state (the transitional state between wakefulness and sleep), mentally recite over and over again with determination and enthusiasm: 'The next time I'm

---

* If you've ever set a strong intent to wake up at a certain hour and succeeded, then you've used exactly the same 'goal-seeking' neurological activation that the MILD technique employs.

** Are you worried that lucid dream training could make you feel less rested? Don't worry, because restorative sleep occurs in delta wave sleep, whereas lucid dreaming is practised in active REM sleep, when the brain is not resting anyway.

dreaming, I'll remember to recognize that I'm dreaming.' Focus on this command and if you feel your mind wandering or realize that it has wandered already, just bring yourself back to the recitation. Totally saturate your mind with the idea. This is the all-important prospective memory and autosuggestion part of the technique and its effectiveness depends on imbuing the recitation with wholehearted 'joyful effort'.*

3. Visualizing lucidity: once you've created and stabilized the strong motivation to *remember to recognize that you're dreaming,* the next step is to visualize yourself back in the dream that you recalled earlier. Really try to relive it in as much detail as you can, envisaging yourself back in it and experiencing it with all your senses as you drift off to sleep. However, this time, imagine that you recognize that you're dreaming and become fully lucid. How? By imagining yourself spotting a dream sign or doing a reality check and then having the realization *Aha! I'm dreaming!*

Then imagine acting out what you might like to do once you're lucid.

The two core principles of the technique are engaging your prospective memory with strong intent and then visualizing yourself getting lucid.

4. Drop off to sleep or do it again: now you can either just fall asleep or repeat steps 2 and 3 again until you feel sure that you've fully engaged the technique, at which point you can drop the technique and allow yourself to fall asleep. In your next dream period, your prospective memory system will become engaged and you will become lucid.

* * *

* One of the Buddhist six perfections, joyful effort is the term used to describe enthusiastic effort for spiritual practice.

> **Charlie says** 💬
>
> *'An easy way to remember the order of this technique is like this: M-I-L-D:*
> *M = Memorize the dream you were just having; I = set the Intent; L =*
> *visualize Lucidity; D = drop off to sleep or do it again.'*

THE 'WAKE UP, BACK TO BED' METHOD

This technique was first posited in the late 1970s by G. Scott Sparrow, the author of *Lucid Dreaming: Dawning of the Clear Light*; it is one of the most effective lucid dreaming techniques available. Research shows that 'wakefulness interjected during sleep increases the likelihood of lucidity'[14] and that this technique is one of 'the most powerful, promising means of achieving lucidity with over two-thirds of participants recording lucid dreams under these circumstances'.[15] In fact, Buddhist scholar B. Alan Wallace references research that calculates that this method increases your chances of lucidity by a whopping 2,000 per cent.[16]

So how do we practise this seemingly too good to be true technique? It's simple. Wake up about two or three hours earlier than normal, stay awake for about an hour and then go back to sleep for another hour or two.

Let's Wake Up and Go 🦋🦋 Back to Bed!

1. Set your alarm for about two or three hours earlier than your usual wake-up time.

2. Wake up and get out of bed.

3. Stay awake for about an hour, engaging in any fully wakeful activity. Meditating or reading about lucid dreaming is ideal, but I've found that just about any mindful activity works well. The aim is not to stay drowsy for the 60 minutes but to waken fully – full wakefulness

being a prerequisite for the technique's efficacy. Having said that, drinking double espressos or answering work e-mails might arouse you a bit too much, so be mindful to keep sleep at arm's reach.

4. After about an hour, reset your alarm for at least an hour or two later, return to bed and fall asleep again with the strong intention to gain lucidity.

One of the ways this technique works is by harnessing the phenomenon of REM rebound. (*For more information on REM rebound, see page 181.*) The last two hours of our sleep cycle are when we do most of our dreaming, so if we starve ourselves of this dream time, when we do eventually go back to sleep we course smoothly and deeply into vivid REM sleep. As REM sleep is the playing field for lucidity, we can see how this technique opens up the potential for getting lucid.

Charlie says

'On a few occasions people have asked me if the hour of wakeful activity could be spent having sex. Well, focusing on your strong intent to gain lucidity for the benefit of all beings would be best, but I guess that having sex would be OK. Just be aware that the tendency of some men to fall asleep right after sex means that you need to time it all quite precisely!'

It's worth noting that all of these techniques require sustained practice for them to work, but as long as we're applying them with the correct motivation, lucidity will surely manifest.

As one Tibetan Buddhist nun says, 'When you plant seeds in the garden, you don't dig them up every day to see if they have sprouted yet. You simply water them and clear away the weeds; you know that the seeds will grow in time.'[17]

Mindfulness of Dream
& Sleep Techniques

'First recognize the dream. Use anything that helps – the techniques elucidated by the dream yogis or any of the methods of modern lucid dreaming.... The whole point is to become lucid within the dream so that you have the basis for whatever dream yoga activities you choose to enact.'[1]

B. ALAN WALLACE

Mindfulness of Dream & Sleep both incorporates and goes far beyond the primary goal of simply lucid dreaming, with aims of more holistic and spiritual benefit. It includes a combination of transformative Western and Tibetan Buddhist dreamwork techniques set within a framework of mindfulness meditation and awareness training.

By combining Western and Eastern techniques, we can take the ancient power of the Tibetan Buddhist approach to dream work and make it accessible to Western practitioners without any homogenization of the two traditions. It's only once we're lucid that the divergence between the lucid dreamer and the dream yogi occurs, so the actual techniques used to reach lucidity can come from either tradition.

Mindfulness of Dream & Sleep practices aim to train our mindful awareness during all stages of dream, sleep and wakefulness. Rather than just focusing on lucid dreaming, we focus on strengthening lucidity in all areas of life, just as the original dream yoga teachings recommend. Fundamentally, Mindfulness of Dream & Sleep is about 'knowing what is happening as it's happening' and developing the power of recognition in all states of experience.

The following practices show us how to wake up to the dream of life as well as the dream of the night and help us to train in lucid living as well as lucid dreaming.

Charlie says

'My teacher Rob Nairn and I created the Mindfulness of Dream & Sleep approach as a way to fill the gap left between the limited scope of Western lucid dreaming practices and the often inaccessible Tibetan dream yoga practices. Mindfulness of Dream & Sleep is for people who want to go beyond lucid dreaming into something much deeper.'

MINDFULNESS MEDITATION

'Just mindfulness. If you train in mindfulness you will surely recognize the dream.'[2] Akong Tulku Rinpoche

Mindfulness meditation is the original lucid dream induction technique and it forms the foundation of all the Mindfulness of Dream & Sleep practices that we're going to explore here.

For thousands of years people have known that training in mindful awareness during the daytime naturally leads to mindful awareness during the night-time and so if we are serious about being lucid in our dreams then meditation practice is a must.

Mindfulness meditation can be practised by people of all faiths and is based on the simple aspiration of 'know what's happening, as it is happening, without preference'. Although many people may find that sitting still in silence is the easiest way to engage this instruction, we can actually practise mindfulness in every action that we perform, whether we are eating, walking, sitting or, of course, dreaming. As long as we 'know what is happening as it is happening, without preference' we are practising mindfulness. It's deceptively simple.

Training ourselves to 'know what is happening as it's happening' will naturally help us to develop the ability to 'know we are dreaming as we're dreaming'. The dream yoga masters tell us that lucid dreaming is dependent on our ability to maintain focused awareness and the ability to 'hold one's mind in check' as we sleep, two qualities directly fostered by mindfulness practice.

Let's look a little more deeply into what mindfulness actually is. We can view our mind as a house and view mindfulness as the tenant of that house. Nobody can enter the house unless the mindful tenant opens the door to them. The tenant is very welcoming and even if an angry thought comes to the door and wants to get in, they won't turn them away or shut them out. In fact they will open the door to the angry thought, listen to it and then simply allow it to leave. At no point does the tenant start chatting to or arguing with the angry thought; they simply allow it in, let it say its piece and then politely show it to the door.

Some people think that meditation is about stopping thoughts, letting the mind go blank or having ecstatic experiences, but mindfulness isn't like that, it is simply about being aware of what is happening in our mind, without preference or judgement.

The French philosopher Blaise Pascal said, 'All of man's misery derives from his inability to sit still, alone, in silence.' So I believe he would have been a firm fan of the following technique.

Any form of mindfulness meditation practice can be used to help fill the lucidity tank, but if you don't have a regular meditation practice already then you might like to try this wonderfully concise mindfulness exercise based on the Mindfulness Association UK's 'Settling, Grounding, Resting with Support' technique:

Let's Do Nothing!

- Sit on a hard-backed chair or on a cushion cross-legged on the floor. Make sure that you're comfortable and have your back straight.*

- First, *settle* the mind by focusing in a very relaxed way on your breath. Breathe in a little more deeply than normal and then gently release the breath.

- You might like to keep in- and out-breaths equal in length, breathing in to a count of three or four and breathing out to a count of three or four.

- If possible, keep your eyes open, but if you would rather close them that's fine, too.

- When you have thoughts, just let them go freely, without attempting to reject or engage them. Simply leave them alone and guide your focus back to the breathing and counting.

- After a few minutes, begin to focus a little more on the out-breath and drop the counting. Notice that as you release the out-breath the body relaxes a little. This is how you settle the mind.

- Now you *ground* the mind in the body by dropping any regulation of the breath** and bringing your focus onto your body. Simply

---

* Western science thinks that sitting up straight is good for you, too. Professor Richard Wiseman cites scientific studies that show how sitting with a straight back leads to an increase in both happiness and mathematical ability.[3]

** The only time you regulate the breath and count is during the settling stage. By lightly regulating the breath, you are working with the respiratory system and coming into an awareness of a hitherto automatic process.

become aware of all the bodily sensations being experienced, that's all.

- You might find that a systematic scanning of the body works well for this. To do this, scan your awareness throughout your body, quite slowly, starting from your feet and ending at your head, then return to the feet and do it again.

- Alternatively, you might choose simply to sit and allow bodily sensations to command your attention as they arise. Becoming aware of the contact points of your body on the floor or seat and noticing any points of bodily tension or relaxation works well.

- Become aware of how your body is supported by the ground beneath you. Feel the weight of your body creating pressure where you're sitting. Let go into the unconditional support of the ground. Be aware of how gravity roots you.

- Once you've scanned your body or allowed your attention to be aware of particular sensations, then become aware of your whole body as it sits in space. Hold your entire body within your awareness.

- Allow yourself to experience how your body exists in space and is surrounded by space. This is how you ground the mind in the body.

- Once you have grounded the mind in the body for about five to ten minutes, move on to resting. You *rest* the mind by letting go of any sense of focus on the body or the breath. Simply rest. Don't try to meditate, just sit there. Give up any idea of trying to do anything. Simply be aware and in touch with whatever comes to you, with a panoramic awareness.

- The point of resting is to allow the mind to relax deeply and to let go of any sense of striving, struggling or trying to achieve. It is not directed in any way, but involves simply being in the moment.

- See if you can rest in this way for one or two minutes at first. This is the highest form of meditation – a flash of the mind's natural unlimited openness. Because our minds are very unsettled, this state is usually very elusive to us. However, here we momentarily taste this freedom, so we sense its possibility.

- When you notice that your mind is becoming involved with thoughts (which might happen after just a few seconds), you can move on to *resting with sound as the support*.

- There are many mindfulness supports you could use, such as the breath or bodily sensations, but I've found that sound is a particularly accessible support for most people.

- For sound to become the support for your mindfulness, simply focus your attention on any and all the sounds that you can hear. Allow sound to anchor your awareness in the present moment.

- Don't reject or engage any of the sounds you can hear, just open up to whatever sounds are naturally present around you: cars outside, footsteps in the next room, the rustling of your clothes, even your own heartbeat.

- Try to hear rather than listen. Listening is often goal-driven and preferential, whereas hearing is more relaxed and open. Just hear and be aware of sound.

- Whenever you drift away into thought and realize, *Oh, I am thinking!*, just very gently, with kind patience and without irritation, return your attention to sound. Remind yourself that there is nothing wrong, that your distracted mind is giving you an opportunity to exercise your muscle of mindfulness, that's all.

- Just sit there, knowing (and hearing) what is happening while it is happening, and each time you drift off, gently bring your mind back to the awareness of sound. Spend about 10 to 15 minutes on resting the mind like this with sound as the support.

· ·

The above practice might take between 20 to 30 minutes, but if you want to, you can extend it for as long as you like, spending the greater portion of it in the 'resting' and 'resting with support' stages.

Top Tips for Mindfulness Meditation

• This practice can be done at any time of day or night, but if you can do it just before bed, all the better for lucid dreaming. The great dream yogi Tenzin Rinpoche says that there is the potential for 'the entire night to be a deep meditation, but it requires a preparation of about 20 minutes before bed'.[4] So, be sure to brush your teeth, let the dog out or do whatever needs to be done before you start your bedtime mindfulness session.

• Never try to stop your thoughts when you meditate. Although you don't want to engage in 'thinking' as such, thoughts will always be part of your mind, just as waves are part of the sea. They aren't something that needs to be subdued, 'rather they are direct expressions of mind's pure, luminous nature'.[5]

• You might like to infuse your meditation with the intention to gain lucidity within your dreams by thinking before you start, *As I train in my capacity for mindful awareness, may I also train in my capacity for lucidity, for the benefit of all beings.** By doing this you are saturating your meditative mind with the intention to gain awareness within your dreams.

• Likewise, at the end of your session, be sure to dedicate the beneficial energy that you will naturally have generated to being more mindfully aware in both your waking life and dreams, for the benefit of all beings.

• Then, once you get up from your seat or cushion, try to maintain the flavour of the meditation and the intention to be more mindfully aware as you continue with your day or prepare for sleep.

---

* It has been scientifically proven that working for the benefit of others also benefits you. When we help others, the two ancient happiness regions of the brain (the *caudate nucleus* and the *nucleus accumbens*) become stimulated, making us feel happy.

WALKING MEDITATION

For those readers who are kinetic learners, it is worth noting that meditation doesn't have to involve sitting still. I spent over ten years working in the professional breakdance scene and I would often see the one-pointed concentration and mindful awareness of meditation being displayed by the b-boys as they spun on their heads. Don't worry, I'm not going to suggest that you all start breakdancing, but those of you who do like to move might like to try walking meditation.*

Walking meditation is a simple but profound practice** and just as easy to learn as sitting meditation. There are many different ways to do it, but here's one of my favourites:

Let's Walk!

- Choose a straight path or flat area about 15 to 20 steps long and simply walk mindfully and slowly from one end of it to the other, turn around and walk back.

- As you walk, centre your gaze at a 45-degree angle in front of you (with your eyes open of course!) and direct your attention to your feet. Focus on the sensation of your feet connecting with the ground.

- Just as you use sound as the support in mindfulness meditation, here you use the sensations in your feet and body as your support as you walk.

- Be fully aware of every feeling that arises from walking. Really enter into the feeling of taking each step – your foot lifting, passing through space and then making contact again with the ground as you move forward.

---

* For something somewhere between the two, I would recommend trying the wonderful combination of dance, movement and meditation that the *School of Movement Medicine* offers.

** When we walk we usually do so with some goal in mind, either to get from A to B or for exercise. Walking mediation, however, has no goal. This allows our overused goal orientation system some well-needed rest.

- Let your posture be upright but relaxed. Let your hands hang by your sides or clasp them gently in front of you. See if you can avoid lapsing into a stroll or amble and can maintain full awareness of every movement you make.

- Experiment with pace; some people like waking really slowly, others at a faster pace, but don't rush, take your time. You might like to regulate your breathing in time with each step, too, but take it nice and slow.

- As you walk, try to open up your senses to the whole experience of walking. While maintaining a primary focus on the sensations of your feet, you can also engage a broad panoramic awareness of the environment in which you are walking.

- Try and practise for 10 or 15 minutes when you first begin and then gradually increase your practice time as you wish.

Charlie says

'I love walking meditation. It's such a great way to integrate mindfulness into your everyday life because after you've been practising it for a while it seeps naturally into your everyday walking habits. You find yourself lightly guiding your breath to the rhythm of your footsteps as you walk to the shops. It even changes the way you dance and the way you run!'

THE STAGES OF SLEEP

Having a basic knowledge of the stages of sleep is fundamental to the Mindfulness of Dream & Sleep approach. We need to be mindful of how we sleep if we want to be mindful while we dream. If we want to dream lucidly then we need to understand when we're most likely to be dreaming, so that we can schedule our lucid dreaming practice accordingly.

Nowadays sleep is broken up into four parts or stages.* Three of the four stages are described in terms of what they are not: non-rapid eye movement or NREM, with dreaming sleep given the honour of being the only one described in terms of what it is: REM. It seems as though dreaming is the main event.

NREM1 or N1 is very light sleep, experienced as drowsiness and often accompanied by alpha brainwave patterns of relaxed wakefulness. The most recognizable aspect of NREM1 sleep is the hypnagogic imagery: the dreamy hallucinations that flash and fade before our mind's eye as we drift off to sleep. As we enter NREM1, we might also experience sudden spasms, known as 'myoclonic jerks',** which will often become incorporated into the hypnagogic 'micro-dreams' somehow, perhaps as stepping off a kerb or falling off a ledge.

As we slip further into sleep, we move from the hypnagogic NREM1 to the complete blackout of NREM2 or N2, in which our heart rate starts to slow and we experience the dissolution of external conscious awareness. We are now asleep. After this blackout, once our brain begins producing delta waves, we are said to have entered NREM3 or N3, stage 3 non-REM sleep, the deepest level of sleep.

This deep delta-wave sleep is restorative sleep. It is the state in which we release HGH (human growth hormone), repair our cells and recharge the batteries. If you manage to wake somebody from the deep delta-wave blackout of NREM3, they will commonly feel groggy and disorientated.

When we first fall asleep, this initial progression from NREM1 to NREM3 takes about half an hour or so. After hanging out in

---

* Sleep scientists used to speak of five stages of sleep, but in 2007 the American Academy of Sleep Medicine decided to group NREM3 and NREM4 together, making four stages.

** Research indicates that these could be the body's response to a lower level of respiration, which the brain occasionally misinterprets as a sign of death and responds with a physical jerk to stimulate it back to life.

NREM3 for about half an hour, we travel back up into NREM2, but then, rather than continuing back to NREM1, we enter a new stage of sleep. Our eyes begin to display rapid movement (REM), our body becomes paralysed and we begin to dream. Dreaming is an active sleep state; we are not resting while we dream. In fact our brains are often more active during dreaming than they are while we are awake.

Our first dream period is only about ten minutes long, and the whole cycle, from falling asleep to the end of our first REM period, usually takes about 90 minutes. We repeat this 90-minute cycle multiple times throughout the night, spending increasingly more time in REM and less time in delta wave as the night progresses. As our REM periods get longer, the last two hours of our night's sleep end up consisting of a majority of REM dreaming. The REM cycle has grown from about 10 minutes to at least 45 minutes or more by the end of an average seven- or eight-hour sleep cycle.

The most important point for lucid dreamers to remember is that the first half of the night is mainly NREM deep sleep with short dream periods and the second half of the night is when we have long REM dream periods with not much entry into deep sleep.

The last few hours of our sleep cycle are also when we will enter dreams most easily from the waking state. This makes it prime time for lucid dreaming. While you can have lucid dreams in the first few hours of your sleep cycle, the dream periods will be short and your mind may be quite groggy. However, in the last few hours you will not only have longer dream periods but you will also have a fair few hours of sleep under your belt, so your mind will feel fresh and ready to engage lucidity.

From a Tibetan Buddhist perspective it is said that clarity dreams (which include lucid dreams) occur more readily in the last two hours of our sleep cycle, so it seems that the last two hours of sleep are really the golden time for lucidity.

Charlie says

'Remember, although the majority of people may sleep in the way described above, you may not be part of that majority. Some people have full-on lucid dreams within 30 minutes of falling asleep at night, but the sleep research says they shouldn't even be dreaming until 80 minutes of sleep have passed. We all sleep differently, so get to know the way that you sleep, not the way everybody else sleeps.'

THE CLEAR LIGHT OF SLEEP

Tibetan Buddhism agrees with the Western scientific view of the four stages of sleep, but the major difference is that the Tibetan tradition views dreamless delta-wave sleep as the most important stage, because it is here that we can experience the clear light of sleep. This essentially occurs when we become super-lucid within the dreamless delta-wave state. It enters us into the state of mind beyond all aspects of subject–object dualism and has been described by the great Tibetan scholar Patrul Rinpoche as 'the original state of the mind, fresh, vast, luminous, and beyond thought'.[6] Clear Light experiences are actually the pinnacle of all dream yoga practice and 'the closest we get to the enlightened mind, where the veils obscuring our enlightened nature are at their thinnest'.[7]

The concept of being lucid within the dreamless void of our own mind is difficult to comprehend, but on the rare occasions that I may have stumbled into the Clear Light of Sleep, I've found it to be an infinite void of what I can only describe as a 'bright darkness', or perhaps more fittingly as a 'dazzling darkness'[8] – a term the early Christian Gnostics used to describe ultimate reality.

So, now that we've explored mindfulness meditation and have an understanding of how our sleep cycles work, let's get back to learning how to become lucid while we sleep.

FAC (FALLING ASLEEP CONSCIOUSLY) INTO DREAM AND SLEEP

This practice combines elements of the well-known Wake Initiated Lucid Dream (WILD) technique with a few of my own conscious sleeping methods and a twist of Buddhist mindfulness. Its aim is to enter either dreamless NREM2 or REM dreaming sleep without blacking out or losing conscious awareness. It is incredibly simple but often quite elusive – letting your body and brain fall asleep while part of your mind stays aware.

FAC into Dream

If you want to enter the dream state consciously from your first descent into sleep at night you will need to maintain conscious awareness throughout all the stages of sleep (N1 to N2 to N3 to REM), which will take most people about 90 minutes in total. Retaining one-pointed awareness for 90 minutes into sleep is a pretty tall order – in fact the Dalai Lama says that 'going through this transition [from wakefulness into sleep] without blacking out is one of the highest accomplishments for a yogi'.[9] Luckily, there is a way that we can cheat a little bit…

If we practise this technique *after briefly waking in the last few hours of our sleep cycle*, we will enter REM dreaming straight from the hypnagogic state – N1 into REM – rather than having to go through the whole sleep cycle again. This means that we can enter REM dreaming within about 15 minutes, which is a much more realistic amount of time to stay conscious and an accomplishment that even L-plate dream yogis can achieve.

For now we'll explore three of the best variations of this technique.

Hypnagogic Drop-in

To enter the dream state lucidly, be like a surfer. Paddle through the hypnagogic imagery and 'drop in' to the wave of the dream lucidly.

Let's Drop In! 🦋🦋

- Sometime after at least four or five hours of sleep, wake up fully and write down your dreams. Then set your intent to gain lucidity, close your eyes and allow yourself to drift back into sleep.

- As you enter N1 sleep, gently focus your mental awareness on the hypnagogic imagery and simply paddle through it, allowing it to build, layer upon layer.*

- The key here is to maintain a delicate vigilance without losing consciousness and being sucked into the dream state unconsciously.

- Try to lead the mind gently into the dream state without blacking out.

- Don't engage the hypnagogic imagery that will arise, but don't reject it either, just lie there watching it until the dreamscape has been formed sufficiently for you to enter it consciously.

- If you feel yourself blacking out, just keep bringing your focus back to the hypnagogic imagery. The imagery is your mindfulness support and is used to keep the thread of your awareness engaged while the rest of you falls asleep.

- The hypnagogic imagery will continue to build layer upon layer until it starts to coalesce into an actual dreamscape. This is a wonderful thing to witness.

---

* Depending on the time of night and varying from person to person, sometimes NREM1 doesn't actually contain much hypnagogic imagery. In that case, simply use the Body and Breath technique instead.

- As the dreamscape solidifies, you might feel a slight pull or sensation of being sucked forward. This is an indication that the wave of the dream is now fully formed. In surfing terms, you are on point-break.

- If you can just stay conscious for a few more moments and are ready to take the plunge, you'll find yourself dropping into the wave of the dream with full lucidity.

Charlie says

'Lucid dreaming is just like surfing. It's all about persistence, balance and movement of energy. Just as we harness the power of the wave to move along it, so we harness the power of the dream. Once we drop into the wave, we don't try to overpower it, we learn to utilize its power to experience something beyond ourselves. It's just the same with dreaming.'

Body and Breath

However far out your mind may seem to go during sleep, there are two aspects of your being that remain in your bed: your body and your breath. In waking meditation we can use the body and the breath as a support to anchor our awareness so that our mind stays stable and is less likely to lose itself in distraction. This is exactly what we want to do as we slip into dream.

Let's Feel!

- Sometime after at least four or five hours of sleep, wake up fully and write down your dreams. Set your intent to gain lucidity, close your eyes and allow yourself to drift back into sleep.

- As you enter sleep, gently focus your mental awareness on the sensations of body and the breath flowing through it.

- The hypnagogic imagery will still arise, but rather than focusing on it as in the hypnagogic drop-in technique, this time focus on your bodily sensations.

- As in the grounding stage of 'Settling, Grounding, Resting with Support', you might find that a systematic scanning of the body works well for this. Alternatively, you might choose to simply allow bodily sensations to command your attention as they arise. Becoming aware of the contact points of your body on the bed works well.

- Once you have scanned your body or allowed your attention to be aware of particular sensations, become aware of your whole body as it lies in space. Hold your entire body within your awareness.

- At some point you may actually feel the body paralysis that accompanies REM sleep setting in. This means that you are on the doorway of the dream.

- If you feel yourself blacking out, just keep bringing your focus back to the sensations of the body and breath. Your mindfulness support is physical sensation.

- By anchoring your awareness in this way you will be able to float through the hypnagogic stage with conscious awareness and enter the dream with full lucidity.

Counting Sleep

By combining counting with constant reflective awareness as you go through the transition from wakefulness into dream, you can maintain your awareness fluidly. This technique is much less meditative than the last two, but is just as effective and some people get the hang of it a bit more easily.

Let's Count Sleep!

- Sometime after at least four or five hours of sleep, wake up fully and write down your dreams. Set your intent to gain lucidity, close your eyes and allow yourself to drift back into sleep.

- As you enter sleep, continuously reflect on your state of consciousness as you count yourself into dreaming, for example, '1. I'm lucid? 2. I'm lucid?' and so on.

- For the first few minutes the answer each time will probably be 'No, I'm still awake!' but once you've counted into the 20s, the answer will probably be 'I am now in the hypnagogic state!'

- If you can make it into the 30s, 40s or even 50s without blacking out, the answer may become 'Almost! The hypnagogic is starting to solidify!'

- Of course the eventual aim is to answer the question with something like '61. I'm lucid? Hang on. Yes, I'm dreaming! I'm lucid!' as you find yourself fully conscious within the dream.*

FAC into Sleep

To use the FAC technique as a conscious sleeping practice, simply apply either the Hypnagogic Drop-in or the Body and Breath techniques as you first fall asleep at night, rather than after four or five hours of sleep. This will allow you conscious access to non-REM sleep.

You might be thinking, *What does non-REM sleep look like?* For many people it is an experience of floating in blackness, because there are no dream projections to fill the space. We are simply a point of disembodied awareness floating in mental potentiality. It sounds quite far out, and preventing yourself from not blacking

---

* Don't count too far beyond 100 though, as by that time you may be too awake for the technique to work.

out as you enter NREM2 can take some practice, but it's well worth it.

Awareness in dreamless sleep is like watching a cinema screen before the projector is turned on: it might not be as exciting as watching the movie, but it shows us that the movie isn't always there. As the late Traleg Rinpoche said, 'The reason that [awareness in] sleep is so potent is that the mind is slowed down, which gives us the opportunity to access the more subtle levels of consciousness we are unable to access during the day.'[10]

Let's Sleep!

- Use the Hypnagogic Drop-in or Body and Breath technique when you first fall asleep at night to drop you into NREM2 rather than REM dreaming.

- As you enter sleep, either gently focus your mental awareness on the hypnagogic imagery or on your bodily sensations.

- Eventually,* the hypnagogic state may fade before blacking out into NREM2. This is the point where we usually lose consciousness and 'fall' asleep.

- If you can maintain consciousness while relaxing into the moment that the hypnagogic state becomes the dreamless sleep state, you will find yourself floating (rather than falling) into non-REM sleep, often as a disembodied point of awareness.

---

* Most people stay in the hypnagogic for about 15 minutes before they enter NREM2. If you are very tired it may only take two minutes, but if you are very alert you can stay in it for hours.

> **Charlie says**
>
> *'Some people wonder how they can tell if they are conscious in the hypnagogic or conscious in non-REM sleep. The hypnagogic is often full of mental imagery and conceptual display, but if you maintain mindfulness throughout it, after 20 minutes or so you come out the other side of it and find yourself in a vast dark space devoid of projections, in which you can no longer feel your body or any sensations of the bed. That is when you're conscious in non-REM sleep – you're consciously sleeping.'*

HYPNAGOGIC AFFIRMATION

This technique requires that you fall asleep while mentally reciting a positive affirmation of your intent to gain lucidity. The hypnagogic state is very similar to the hypnotic state, so if we apply a suggestion or affirmation within it, we may find that it has the potential to work with hypnotic effect.

Within the dream yoga teachings of the great master Guru Rinpoche, it is said that you should 'bring forth a powerful yearning to recognize the dream state',[11] so you really need to make your intent to gain lucidity strong and real for this to work properly. You can do this as you first fall asleep at night or, even better, after an early hours wake-up, but whenever you do, the important thing is to imbue your sleepy consciousness with the fervent aspiration to gain lucidity.

This is one of the most accessible Mindfulness of Dream & Sleep techniques because you can do it every time you fall asleep.

Let's Affirm!

- As you enter the hypnagogic state, continuously recite an affirmation such as 'I recognize my dreams with full lucidity' or 'When I dream, I know that I'm dreaming' or whatever phrase you feel best encapsulates your intention to get lucid.

- It is important to recite your affirmation with heartfelt determination rather than just robotically repeating it till you get bored. Without determination, this technique simply won't work.

- When mentally reciting the affirmation, the important thing is not that you're repeating it right up to the point at which you enter the dream (although that would be best), but more that you saturate your last few minutes of conscious awareness with the strong intention to gain lucidity.

- If you are a spiritual practitioner you could create an affirmation out of the mantra or incantation of an enlightened energy form with whom you feel a connection. For example, I like to use the mantra of Amitabha Buddha (*Om ami dewa hri*) to form part of a rhyming affirmation: '*Om ami dewa hri*, I will have a lucid dream.' This not only serves the purpose of the technique, but it also imbues the practice with the blessing of the mantra.

Charlie says

'When I first practised this technique I used the phrase "I must have a lucid dream" and found that I was getting very tight with the practice and having poor results. Then it hit me: my unconscious is naturally rebellious – it doesn't want to be told that it must do something! So I changed my affirmation to "I love lucid dreaming" and my pleasure-seeking unconscious met my request straightaway!'

NAPPING

When I was in my early 20s I hardly ever took naps. I was far too busy trying to change the world. But now I realize that if you really want to change the world, you should take a nap.

A nap is any short period of sleep outside your main sleep cycle and is one of the most beneficial things that you can do for both your psychological and physiological health. Napping charges your body with potential, and whatever activities you engage in after a nap will be executed more easily and tackled more creatively.

A 2009 Harvard University study has shown that those who nap regularly are 37 per cent less likely to die of heart disease than non-nappers.[12] Heart disease is one of the biggest killers in the Western world and if medical science produced a new pill that could reduce our risk of dying from it by 37 per cent, we'd all be queuing up to buy it. There's no need to queue, just have a snooze!

As well as being great for the body and mind, napping also has a wealth of lucid dreaming benefits. During an afternoon nap, we tend to enter REM dreaming sleep straightaway and to stay there for most of the nap without much entry into delta-wave deep sleep, if any at all.

Chinese Taoist dream practitioners saw from early on that having only one opportunity per day to enter the dream state wasn't enough for serious dream yoga practice and so they made daily napping a central part of their tradition. They realized that by napping during the day, when we entered our full sleep cycle at night our body was already quite rested, so sleep wasn't engaged in out of fatigue but more deliberately for the goal of spiritual practice.[13]

Naps provide great neurological benefits for the lucid dreamer, too. Biological psychologists have discovered that 'habitual nappers' have greater alpha and theta EEG power in stages one and two of sleep,[14] meaning that their brain capacity is actually enhanced throughout REM sleep, thus aiding lucidity. Suddenly an afternoon nap doesn't seem so lazy after all.

Recent studies at the University of Surrey sleep lab have concluded that most British people feel the urge to nap from about 1 p.m. to 3 p.m.[15] and that mid-afternoon is one of the best times to nap based on our circadian rhythms (changes in mental and physical characteristics that occur in the course of a day), but a nap at any point during the day will do the trick.

Try not to nap for more than 60–90 minutes, though, because anything over that may lead you into delta-wave sleep, which might make you feel a bit groggy when you wake up from it. Most people find that a nap of between 20 and 60–90 minutes is best.

New findings about how sleep hormones are released into the body have shown that sleepiness is as regulated by light exposure as it is by actual tiredness.[16] So, if you want to have a nap but feel too lively to get to sleep, you should try avoiding bright lights and be in a darkened environment before you hit the sack. Happy napping!

Let's Nap!

- Remind yourself of the potential that a nap holds: rapid entry into REM sleep, great for lucid dream practice and a good way to refresh your body and mind.
- Go to sleep for between 20 and 60–90 minutes anytime outside your usual sleep cycle and if you like, try to recognize your dreams.

Charlie says

'I was in a lucid dream once when I invoked the presence of the Tibetan master Guru Rinpoche. When he appeared, I asked him, "How can I be of most benefit to all beings?", to which he replied, "Take a nap." I guess I was expecting something a bit more profound, but I've taken his advice to heart nonetheless!'

Going Deeper into Mindfulness of Dream & Sleep

'Relax but do not fall asleep, and be in a state
of awareness for as long as you can.'[1]
DON JUAN MATIS, YAQUI INDIAN SORCERER

Now that we've covered many of the basic lucidity techniques, we'll be moving deeper into the practice of Mindfulness of Dream & Sleep. Remember, Part II of this book is like a toolbox, full of different tools for different jobs, so don't feel that you should be practising every technique every night. A successful practitioner will know their toolbox and select the correct tools for the particular job.

The next tools to look at are the meditative sleeping practices that involve maintaining mindful awareness through the gateways into and out of sleep.

THE HYPNAGOGIC AND HYPNOPOMPIC STATES

As we discussed earlier, the hypnagogic state is the transitional state of mind that lies between wakefulness and sleep. It is the dozy in-between state often characterized by hypnagogic imagery – the visual or often conceptual displays that flash and fade before our mind's eye as we drift off to sleep. These hypnagogic images are made up of memories of the day, mental preoccupations and, for some people, a whole load of crazy shapes, colours and faces. I imagine these eccentric displays of mind as a bit like the flashes of colour that you see during the final moments of a sunset, and, just like those final moments, they offer us a rare glimpse of our own inner light.

At the other end of sleep we find the hypnopompic state, which is the transitional state of mind that lies between sleep and full wakefulness. Most people hardly even notice the hypnopompic state because they pass through it so quickly in their rush to wake up. If only we would spend more time exploring it, we would find that it's a state often characterized by flashes of inspiration and non-judgemental mind as the sun rises afresh out of the darkness of sleep. I call these flashes of clarity 'hypnopompic insights'. If you're interested in the kind of insights that can be gained in this state, check out the hypnopompic insight section in Appendix II (see *page 266*).

The hypnopompic is most commonly experienced as the half-sleep state that we enter into after we've hit the alarm clock's snooze button in the morning. It's the state that we experience just before our mind has woken fully from sleep and when our eyes are still usually closed. It is a subtler state than the hypnagogic and contains much less mental imagery because it's a state of mind in which we are partially awake but are yet to engage in fully conscious thinking.*

The unique feature of the hypnopompic is that because it occurs *after* a period of sustained sleep and dream, it is a much

---

* This doesn't mean that there aren't thoughts in the hypnopompic, but we are much less likely to *engage* the thoughts with our chattering conceptual mind.

more refined state of mind, due to the psychological processing that occurs during sleep and dream.

Both the hypnagogic and the hypnopompic have tremendous potential for psychological growth, but at the same time they each have their pros and cons. If we stick with the rising and setting sun metaphor that I used before, we can see that the hypnagogic might be associated with the diminishing of reflective consciousness as the sun of our awareness sets for the night whereas the hypnopompic might be associated with the emergence of reflective consciousness as the sun of awareness rises after its slumber. The hypnagogic is, of course, characterized by drowsiness, because we are falling asleep, while the hypnopompic is characterized by a soft clarity of mind, because we have just been refreshed by sleep and aren't yet fully awake.

As we learned earlier, mindfulness meditation is about 'knowing what is happening as it is happening', so hypnagogic and hypnopompic mindfulness techniques are about knowing what is happening as it is happening while we're dozing or snoozing. But what are the benefits of staying mindful in these states and how do we actually do it? Let's zzzzzzz...

Hypnagogic Mindfulness (The Tao of Dozing)

We pass through the hypnagogic state every time we fall asleep, which means that we have a daily opportunity to engage it with awareness and even engage mindfully the sleep that it leads us into. It's a state of huge potential, but how can we spend more time in it than the ten or so minutes that it usually takes us to fall asleep? We must learn the Tao of Dozing…

By applying similar techniques to the ones we learned in the Mindfulness Meditation section earlier (see *page 88*), we can literally meditate into sleep, which, as the Buddhist master Mingyur Rinpoche said, 'will mean that the sleep mind forms out of the meditation mind, which will make the sleep a meditation'.[2]

If we can practise mindfulness* within it, the hypnagogic state can contain riches that will make us feel as though we've been sleeping on a goldmine for our whole life but have never gone digging.

This technique is about learning to rest on the drowsy boundary of sleep. The key to it is to be fully aware of the process of falling asleep so that we can begin to slow it down, giving ourselves extended access to the hypnagogic state and even bringing awareness into sleep with us.

This practice can be done at night as a precursor to sleep but is best learned and explored during the daytime, when we are less likely to fall prematurely into full sleep. If we practise it during the day, as an alternative to an afternoon nap, we may find that it refreshes our mind even more effectively than napping. It's a bit like putting the computer into 'hibernate' mode rather than 'shut down' mode: we save our battery power but don't take so long to boot back up again!

Let's Doze!

- After setting an alarm for 20 minutes hence, lie down on your back, with a pillow under your head, and close your eyes. Adjust your body as you like and allow yourself to be comfortable, but not too hot – you don't want to fall asleep, remember!

- Become aware of your breathing and then proceed to settle your mind, ground yourself in your body, rest in awareness and rest with sound as your support. Use the 'Settling, Grounding, Resting with Support' technique that we learned earlier (see page 90), but with the difference that your eyes are closed and you are lying down.

- If hypnagogic imagery (both visual or conceptual) starts to manifest, just be aware of it without engaging with it or rejecting

---

* Hypnagogic mindfulness is very similar to the Yoga Nidra practices and each practice can complement the other.

it. Simply rest in the awareness of the hypnagogic, and if you feel yourself starting to slip into sleep, bring your attention back to the sounds of your breathing and the sounds in the room.

- If you feel that you are about to black out completely, you might like to lightly contract your fingers or toes as a way of bringing yourself back to bodily awareness.
- Allow yourself to rest in mindful awareness of the hypnagogic state for about 20 minutes to begin with. You can extend the time with practice.

After learning and exploring this technique during the daytime, you can apply it at night to form a 'conscious sleeping' technique. After 20 minutes or so, rather than stopping the practice, maintain the same mindful awareness as you transition into sleep.

Charlie says

'My audio CD, Lucid Dreaming, Conscious Sleeping (Hay House) contains a great 20-minute guided hypnagogic mindfulness practice based on this technique.'

Hypnagogic Creativity

The hypnagogic state is a wonderfully creative place in which intuitive ideas flow effortlessly as our brain switches from the linear, logical left-brain dominance of the day to the intuitive, imaginative right-brain dominance of the night. Although hypnagogic imagery may seem to be nothing more than the unintelligible side effect of the brain 'shutting down' ready for sleep, it's actually much more than this.

For hundreds of years, both left- and right-brainers have been using the hypnagogic state as a kind of 'holodeck' for creative problem-solving and thinking outside the box of logical thought.

Its unique combination of right-brain dominance with wakeful awareness makes it the perfect place to see ideas in a new light.

Edison, the inventor of the light bulb, used to engage the hypnagogic state for creative problem-solving and even accredited his final design for the light bulb to a revelation that he had while drifting into a hypnagogic nap.

Each afternoon, Edison would prepare an armchair with two metal plates under the armrests. He would then hold ball bearings in his hands, place them on the armrests and have a nap.[3] As he dozed, the ideas and research that he had been working on would float into his mind and stew in the creative juices of the hypnagogic. When his body entered full sleep, muscle paralysis would set in and the ball bearings in his hands would be released, hit the metal plates below and wake him up, allowing him to jot down any new revelations or ideas.

Salvador Dali was also partial to a bit of hypnagogic roving and would often use his hypnagogia as inspiration for his work, which, when combined with a pint of absinth, presumably led to the 100-foot elephants stepping over melting clocks.

Dali had a slightly different technique, though. He would lie down on a couch and put a glass on the floor. He would then carefully place one end of a spoon on the edge of the glass and the other end in his hand. He would float into the hypnagogic state, mindful of all the imagery, and when his hypnagogic state became full REM dreaming and muscle paralysis set in, he would naturally lose his grip on the spoon, which would crash into the glass noisily enough to wake him. He would then immediately sketch the bizarre hypnagogic imagery that he had witnessed.[4]

More recently, a 2001 Harvard study cited in Deirdre Barrett's *The Committee of Sleep* found proof that the hypnagogic state really was a great place for creative problem-solving. The researchers concluded that although full-blown dreams were great at working with and reflecting upon psychological issues, the hypnagogic state was especially effective at 'problem solving that benefited from hallucinatory images being critically examined while still before the eyes'.[5] This is because hypnagogic imagery can be evaluated consciously as it manifests and so it becomes a much more accessible source of creativity than full-blown dreams, which have to be remembered and often interpreted before their meaning is revealed.

So, let's learn how to use the hypnagogic state for creativity.

Let's Get Creative!

- Set your intent to explore a certain creative task within the hypnagogic state.

- Set an alarm for five to 20 minutes hence, lie down on your back with a pillow under your head and close your eyes. Adjust your body as you like and allow yourself to be comfortable.

- Become aware of your breathing and allow yourself to enter the hypnagogic state. If you want to use the 'Settling, Grounding, Resting with Support' technique (see page 90), then please do, but use your particular creative task as your support rather than sound.

- Once you are resting in the hypnagogic state, engage in the creative task you wish to explore through visualizing it or feeling it out and allowing your right-brain creativity to engage it in a non-linear way.* Use your breath and bodily sensations to ground you if you feel that you are getting too close to full sleep, and be sure to note down any creative insights you've had. Try short bursts of five to ten minutes first, because you don't want to risk falling asleep before you've noted down your creative insights.

---

* If you've been strongly focusing on a certain task or question in the hours before you enter the hypnagogic, it may well surface of its own accord.

Hypnopompic Mindfulness (Snooze Button Meditation)

The hypnopompic state is as creative and imaginative a state as the hypnagogic, but because it occurs after the psychological processing of sleep and dream, it contains a clarity and vastness unmatched by the hypnagogic. Whereas the hypnagogic is characterized by imagery and visuals, the hypnopompic is often more of a blank canvas, a clear, non-conceptual awareness dawning like the sun. By accessing the hypnopompic we are gaining insight into our mind at its clearest and most radiant, as the clutter of the previous day's residues and chattering thoughts has been filed away. For many people, mindfulness meditation applied in the hypnopompic can be one of the most refined experiences of pure consciousness that they have.

My teacher Rob Nairn is a hypnopompic specialist and it was his idea to introduce the practice of hypnopompic mindfulness into the retreats and workshops we were running. Rob actually believes that ·this practice offers the potential 'for a level of profound psychological exploration unmatched by any other state of mind'.[6] He also thinks that it might be even more beneficial than lucid dreaming, because although it can take a while to get to grips with lucid dreaming, you can learn the hypnopompic mindfulness within a couple of sessions.

The hypnopompic state dawns like a vast expanse of awareness after our often cluttered, illogical dreams, and if we can learn to rest within it we will often gain insight into the nature and meaning of the dreams we have just been having with far greater ease than if we were to reflect upon them once fully awake.*

In a nutshell, if you want to tap into your full potential, hit the snooze button.

---

* Ayang Rinpoche says that during sleep the energy of our consciousness collects at the heart centre, where the mind is said to reside. This means that our first thought is particularly important because it infuses the whole mind with its flavour.

Let's Snooze!

- The hypnopompic state can only be entered from full sleep. If you can, try to enter it naturally by allowing yourself to wake up slowly and mindfully in the morning, without opening your eyes if possible. Simply become mindful of that brief space between sleep and wakefulness that you pass through every time you wake up. When you feel yourself waking up and entering this state, don't open your eyes, don't move your body and try not to engage in too much 'thinking' as such – just lie there mindfully aware. The hypnopompic is a vast space in which awareness can naturally rest, so do just that, while remaining mindful of any spontaneous insights that might arise.

- For many of us, entering the hypnopompic naturally can be a bit tricky, due to our habitual use of an alarm clock, but not to worry. If you can't enter it naturally, just set your alarm 10 or 20 minutes before you intend to wake up. Make sure that the alarm is within easy reach, and when it sounds, wake up very gently (without opening your eyes if possible) and hit the 10- or 20-minute snooze button mindfully, not in a rushed, chaotic way.*

- After you've hit the snooze button, lie back down, close your eyes (if you needed to open them to hit the snooze button) and become aware of your breathing. Due to the nature of the hypnopompic, a simple awareness of breath meditation is all that is needed here: simply knowing when you're breathing in and when you're breathing out. If you feel yourself slipping back into sleep, just bring yourself back to the awareness of breath and the feeling of your body being supported by the bed.

5. Allow your mind to rest in the broad panoramic warmth of the hypnopompic state. After 10 or 20 minutes the snooze alarm will sound, and you can either wake up fully or repeat the exercise.

---

* On the retreats I run, I use the high-pitched tone of a singing bowl to bring people out of sleep and into the hypnopompic state, but you could use any sound that rouses you out of sleep.

Charlie says

'The hypnopompic often gets overlooked because it's mistakenly seen as the mind at its bleariest, but this is often just because we haven't had enough sleep preceding it. If we can enter the hypnopompic refreshed and are able to maintain awareness within it, morning grogginess will be a thing of the past and we'll be able to start every morning mindfully aware.'

It should be noted that the enhanced clarity of the hypnopompic also means a lack of self-censorship, which often shines light into the dark corners of our mind and sometimes reveals our deepest fears and neuroses, which we unconsciously repress during our waking hours. But if we can learn to rest in this state with non-judgemental awareness, simply witnessing, we will naturally begin to integrate these neuroses into the wholeness of ourselves. As the great Krishnamurti once said, 'The seeing is the doing.'[7]

Insomniacs often spend a lot of time in the hypnopompic in the middle of the night, as they wake up after a few hours of slumber and then can't get back to sleep. This is a state often referred to as 'the 4 a.m. demons', but it's actually a beacon of light in a night of sleeplessness. Most people reject it, fearing it out of habit, whereas in fact this process is part of the wonderfully beneficial hour of the wolf…

THE HOUR OF THE WOLF

It's 4 a.m. and you're wide awake. Perhaps you've been asleep since you hit the sack a few hours ago or perhaps you've hardly slept yet, but right now it seems as though everybody else in the whole world is asleep and you're awake. It's a disaster. You're abnormal. You're messed up. You're an insomniac. You're a freak.

No, you're not a freak – you're a wolf.

The hour of the wolf is what millions of people could appreciate and experience with fascination if they could only drop the expectation that they should be asleep during it. In fact I am writing this paragraph at 4:10 a.m., feeling full of ideas and inspiration. While the world sleeps, my mind feels fresh and creative. The 4 a.m. demons are waiting in the wings, but I know that they feed off anxiety, so as long as I don't throw meat into their den they'll stay placated and inactive. In fact I might go and visit them later on.

Jeff Warren, author of *Head Trip*, the wonderfully researched travelogue of the human mind, believes that waking at this time of night, which he calls 'the Watch', is actually a very natural phenomenon that harks back to our pre-industrial sleep cycle. Yes, that's right, before the 1800s – and thus for a much longer period of human history – people slept very differently.

Before the early 1800s most people in northern Europe and Britain, plus many in countries under the control of the British Empire, slept in two bouts. Allowing for seasonal fluctuations, the first bout was usually from about 9 p.m. to midnight and the second bout was from about 2 a.m. to dawn. So what happened between midnight and 2 a.m.? People were wide awake and doing stuff! They might go and check on their cows in the fields or they might go to a friend's place and have a drink, they might have sex, but whatever they chose to do, one thing is for certain – they would be wide awake.

We slept in that way for thousands of years and our new way of sleeping (six to eight hours in one go) is still in the experimental phase. This means that the 'freaks' and 'insomniacs' who are wide awake in the early hours might simply be displaying a much more natural and ancient sleep cycle than the rest of us. Perhaps it's those who strive for eight hours of uninterrupted sleep who are the real freaks!

Buddhist teachers agree with Warren, saying, 'Human beings have been hardwired from prehistoric times to spend a good portion of their nocturnal hours in a resting state that lies somewhere between wakefulness and sleep.'[8] But one question remains: what happened in the early 1800s to change the sleeping pattern we'd had for thousands of years?

The industrial revolution happened. Warren tells us that three developments that accompanied it soon came to affect the sleeping patterns of Londoners, and with London being the centre of the industrialized world, the sleeping patterns of much of humanity. Coffee, affordable books and light bulbs were, along with the factory owners' desire to work their employees for longer hours, three of the contributing factors that changed the way we slept, because people could stay awake longer, tanked up on caffeine, reading affordable novels by the light of an electric bulb. Who would have thought that three seemingly unrelated developments could combine to affect our lives so dramatically, without us even realizing it?

Charlie says

'However you sleep, the important thing to remember here is that if you are someone who wakes in the middle of the night and feels unable to go back to sleep, don't fret – you might be displaying a much more natural sleeping pattern than the rest of us.'

Nobody sleeps for eight solid hours, however much it may seem that way. Sleep is a constant state of flux, moving tidally throughout the night, coursing from the shallows to the depths. David Neubauer, author of *Understanding Sleeplessness*, says: 'Thinking it's necessary to stay asleep for eight hours straight may be unrealistic… but since we're conditioned to think that waking during the night is a problem, when it happens we panic, a reaction that causes our brains to awaken even further.'[9]

Multiple wake-ups throughout the night are fine, too, and even waking every 60 to 90 minutes can be part of a healthy sleep pattern. We sleep in 90-minute cycles, so brief wakenings after each cycle as we work our way back up through the sleep stages are natural and don't affect our sleep detrimentally. In fact, as part of my research into bringing mindful awareness into every moment of my sleep and dream cycle, I have on occasion tried to be aware of each of these 90-minute trips to the surface, even briefly opening my eyes to check the time so that in the morning I have a rough approximation of the timings of every one of the four or five sleep and dream cycles that occur throughout my eight-hour sleep. And yes, I wake up feeling just as refreshed.

Most of us do have brief awakenings throughout the night, but because we ordinarily don't have any memory of them, we think we've slept constantly. Insomniacs, however, because of their hyper-conscious fear of not being able to sleep when they should be asleep, tend to grasp at these micro-awakenings to fuel the negative expectation that they 'should' be asleep, and so perpetuate the cycle.

If you do find that you wake up in the early hours and can't get back to sleep, just drop any expectation of sleeping and definitely don't try to fall asleep.* Instead, either practise hypnopompic mindfulness (especially if you class yourself as an insomniac) or simply enjoy the cortically rich, alert clarity of the hour of the wolf and use it creatively, as I am doing right now as I type this paragraph into my phone.

---

* Rob Nairn once told me, 'Insomnia is trying to fall asleep.'

THE MULTIPLE WAKE-UPS TECHNIQUE

We now know that we have multiple micro-awakenings each night, but how we can use these to aid lucidity? It's simple: if we fall asleep once a night and then wake up once in the morning, we are only giving ourselves one opportunity to engage Mindfulness of Dream & Sleep. That's just one opportunity to fall asleep consciously, one opportunity to recall our dreams and one opportunity to engage the lucid dreaming techniques. But if we wake ourselves up and fall back to sleep three times a night then we triple our potential success rate!

On the Mindfulness of Dream & Sleep retreats that I run we have our first wake-up about four or five hours after going to sleep and then do two or three more alarmed wake-ups 90 minutes or so hence. The first few hours of sleep are when we get most of our deep restorative sleep, so we don't interrupt that, but the second few hours, as you'll remember, are when we start to have longer dream periods, with the last two hours of our sleep cycle being the prime time for dreaming. And don't worry, if we time the wake-ups to coincide with our ascent into the upper regions of sleep (which occur at the end of every 90-minute sleep cycle), then we won't feel any less rested the next day.

The multiple wake-ups technique has been used by Tibetan dream yogis for hundreds of years and in the dream yoga teachings of Namgyal Rinpoche we are actually instructed: 'Instead of a long continuous sleep, try to sleep for short periods by deliberately waking yourself up in order to review whether you have successfully recalled or recognized your dream.'[10]

Let's Wake Up!

A typical night-time schedule on a Mindfulness of Dream & Sleep retreat goes like this. After an initial period of about five hours of sleep alone in our beds (three 90-minute cycles plus 30 minutes leeway), we wake up and go to the meditation hall, where we have a 'sacred sleeping area' set up. Then, once we are side by side with our fellow dreamers, the night progresses in 90-minute sessions interspersed with periods of up to ten minutes for dream documentation. This process greatly increases the chances of having a lucid dream and I recommend all dreamwork practitioners try it.

Feel free to adapt the schedule below to suit your personal sleep cycle and waking times. Experiment, be brave and see what works for you.

- 11 p.m.–4 a.m: First session of sleep and dreams, with focus on restful deep sleep rather than any dream work *per se.*

- 4 a.m.–5:30 a.m: Second session of sleep and dreams, with specific lucid dream induction methods (e.g. the FAC technique).

- 5:40 a.m.–7:10 a.m: Third session of sleep and dreams, with specific lucid dream induction methods (e.g. the MILD technique).

- 7:20 a.m.–8:20 a.m: Fourth session of sleep and dreams, with specific lucid dream induction methods (e.g. the Hypnagogic Affirmation technique).

- 8:20 a.m.–8:35 a.m: Hypnopompic mindfulness practice (lights on).

This schedule gives you over eight hours of sleep, 15 minutes of snooze meditation and triples the chance of getting lucid each night!

You might even like to think about setting up your own sacred sleeping area in your home. The simple act of dividing your sleep into a period of rest in bed followed by a period of spiritual practice (in a place other than your bed) creates a powerful energetic intent that directly translates into lucidity.

THE 4, 7, 8 BREATH

While practising the Multiple Wake-ups technique some people find that they get so energized by anticipation of their next wake-up that they have trouble getting back to sleep.

So far we've explored several mindfulness meditation techniques that can be applied during our sleeping hours to help improve our clarity, but not yet explored one that actually helps us to fall asleep. This is where the 4, 7, 8 Breath comes in.

The 4, 7, 8 Breath is a natural tranquilliser for the nervous system. But unlike tranquillizing drugs, which often lose their power over time, this exercise gains in power with repetition and practice.[11]

Dr Andy Weil, one of the most vocal proponents of this technique, says, 'This is a great way to help you fall asleep. If you wake up in the middle of the night and can't get back to sleep, this technique will help you fall asleep right away.'[12]

. . . .

Let's Breathe!

- Sitting on your bed ready for sleep, place your tongue behind your upper front teeth and exhale completely and audibly through your mouth.

- Now close your mouth and inhale through your nose for four counts.

- Next, hold your breath for seven counts.
- Finally, release your breath through your mouth audibly for eight counts.
- Repeat this process just four times for the first few times you do it, then increase your repetitions as you like up to 12 times.
- This is a form of yogic breathing and it's very good for your overall health as well as being a great insomnia tool.

Charlie says

'Another great tip for getting back to sleep mindfully during the Multiple Wake-ups technique comes from Tibetan medicine. Drinking hot water at about 4 a.m., the time when the subtle energies are said to enter the central energy system, not only helps us sleep better but also invites the subtle energies to flow correctly, which helps us get lucid.'

DREAM AWARENESS PRACTICE

Not all dreams are laden with mystical meaning – sometimes they are simply the mind filing through the past day's memories – but occasionally we all experience a dream that we know beyond doubt contains an energy of insight or revelation. It's with these dreams that we practise Dream Awareness.

When we interpret dreams consciously, we often try to replace the dream's intelligence with our own, but instead we should listen to, and hear, with broad awareness, the tone of the dream, satisfied in the knowledge that we will be shown what we need to be shown. Our dreams don't conceal their meaning from us, it's just that we often don't understand their language. Just like us, a dream wants to be understood, not interpreted or rationalized, and to understand a dream we must offer it our attentive awareness.

As I mentioned in Chapter 3, our rational mind needs to drop its expectations and linear logic if it wants to understand what the unconscious mind is offering. If we want to gain an awareness of a dream's potential insight then we need to bathe in its underlying energy rather than trying to interpret it directly, symbol by symbol. This process of soaking in the flavour of the dream will allow any insight to arise spontaneously, without the rational mind jumping to conclusions or creating false meaning.

From a Buddhist point of view, 'many of our dreams are not actually worth interpreting',[13] due to the belief that they most commonly arise from the deluded mindstream, and yet becoming aware of our dreams (rather than interpreting them) is seen as beneficial.* The dream yogis say, 'When we become aware of our dreams we will start waking up to our delusory thoughts while we are awake… we will stop being duped by our fantasies.'[15]

Dream Awareness is a Mindfulness of Dream & Sleep practice rather than a lucid dreaming practice as such, but I encourage all lucid dreamers to adopt it nonetheless. To make a conscious effort to get in touch with the feeling of a dream, to spend some time in its emotional flavour (rather than just recalling its content), is to spend time hanging out with your unconscious, paying homage to its offerings and familiarizing yourself with its ways – just the kind of things lucid dreamers need to be doing as much as they can!

••

Let's Be Aware! 🦋

Upon waking from a vividly recalled dream, lie there, eyes open, in wakeful awareness (or return to the shallows of the hypnopompic if you like) and bring the dream to mind.

---

* There are no dream dictionaries in Tibetan Buddhism, but Tibetan medicine does engage in some dream interpretation. Apparently 'to dream of riding backwards on a donkey while naked might indicate to the doctor the death of a patient.'[14]

Rest in awareness with the dream as your support. You don't have to visualize yourself back in it as such, but try to bring forth its main flavour and essence.

Without falling back asleep, allow yourself to soak in the underlying feeling of the dream. Try not to interpret or rationalize its content or search for meaning. Simply lie there and allow any insights to arise spontaneously with a non-preferential acceptance.

If you want a more structured approach to Dream Awareness, you can apply the RAIN technique to the dream. RAIN stands for 'Recognize, Allow, Intimate attention, Non-identification' and is a great mindfulness meditation technique that I first learned through the Mindfulness Association UK.

Let It RAIN!

To apply RAIN within the Dream Awareness practice, awaken from a vividly recalled dream and lie there, eyes open, in wakeful awareness (or in the hypnopompic state) and bring the dream to mind, Then simply:

- *Recognize* a core element of the dream.
- *Allow* its underlying flavour to arise without judgement and provide a friendly space for it.
- *Intimately* attend to the aspect of the dream without trying to interpret it directly. Then finally try to engage…
- *Non-identification:* be mindful not to identify with whatever arises but simply accept it as it is.

Mindfulness Association instructor Fay Adams says, 'The non-identification stage can be hard to get a feel for at first. What we are doing is taking a few steps back so that we see all that we've been recognizing, allowing and giving our intimate attention to as part of a bigger picture. We zoom out and see that this is one aspect of our experience, not all that we are. This may allow the core element of the dream to express itself on its own terms or dissolve away.'*

> **Charlie says**
>
> 'Dream awareness is a great way to understand our dreams without limiting them through direct translation. It allows the underlying meaning of a dream to arise without censorship or rationalization, meaning that we get to know our dreams in their full character on their own terms.'

PRAYER

'When about to sleep, pray that you may be enabled to comprehend the dream state and firmly resolve that you will comprehend it.'
TIBETAN DREAM YOGA TEACHINGS OF NAROPA

I know that just by mentioning the 'P' word I may cause some readers to skip forward to the next chapter, but hang about for a bit while I explain. Prayer is one of the most effective lucid dreaming techniques that I have ever come across, so it would do this book a disservice not to look into it.

When I talk of prayer, it's not quite as you might imagine. Perhaps when we pray it's not just that some external God or Buddha is answering our prayers, but actually that unconsciously our own divine Buddha nature directs our behaviour to become congruent with the actions necessary to achieve the goals of these prayers. By praying for a specific change in ourselves, we begin to create a powerful new habit that will eventually lead to the manifestation of the change that we have prayed for. In short,

---

* For more instruction on using RAIN within meditation, check out the courses offered by the Mindfulness Association UK.

it's not just the exterior deity who answers our prayers, it's our own enlightened nature.

I've found that when people of faith spend a few minutes before bed praying for lucidity to their personal embodiment of enlightenment, be it the Buddha, Jesus, Allah, the universe or even their own higher self, it can be more effective than all the scientifically verified lucidity techniques put together. Once we magnify our focused intent through the power that these enlightened archetypes exert, it becomes much more than just 'hoping to get lucid'.

Prayer was one of my sticking points when I first encountered Buddhism at the age of 17. The Buddha refused to acknowledge any God or creator deity outside ourselves, and initially I had been attracted to Buddhism partly due to this, but then once I got into it I found that I was being asked to pray all the time. *Pray to whom? Pray for what?* I thought. Then I found out that in Tibetan Buddhism we don't pray to a creator God or an external divinity, but to the enlightened potential that resides within us all, either through external personifications of enlightenment in the form of buddhas, enlightened archetypes and great masters or the internal potential of Buddha nature inherent in all sentient beings. In Buddhism, what is important is not to whom you pray but the devotion of the prayer itself.*

It started making a bit more sense to me, but then one day I came across the well-known 'Story of the Dog's Tooth' and it all became crystal clear. Here it is in my own words...

There was once an old and very devoted Buddhist woman who lived in Tibet with her only son. The son was a silk merchant who often made trips to northern India to trade his wares. Each time he went to India his mother would plead with him

---

* In *59 Seconds*, Professor Richard Wiseman cites a study from the University of Michigan suggesting that praying for other people may be as good for your health as praying for yourself.[16]

to bring her back a Buddhist relic or holy object which she could place on her shrine to help inspire her prayers, but each time he refused her request. After decades of pleading, the old woman (who was now as stubborn as she was old) told her son that if he didn't get her some sort of Buddhist relic or holy object, she would kill herself!

The son placated his mother and promised that he would fulfil her wish, but the next time that he travelled to India he returned to Tibet empty-handed. In fact he had been so busy with selling his silk that he had completely forgotten about his promise and only remembered his mother's threat when he turned down the path that led to their house. In a fit of panic he scanned the path for ideas and saw the rotting corpse of a dog by the side of the road. In a flash of desperate inspiration he pulled out one of the teeth from the corpse, wrapped it in a piece of his finest silk and decided to present it to his mother as the tooth of Buddha himself, one of the holiest Buddhist relics in existence.

His mother met him at the door with a face that told him that she was ready to keep her suicidal promise, so he swiftly presented her with the tooth and an elaborate tale of how he had come across it. The old woman was ecstatic and rushed over to her small shrine, where she carefully placed the deceased dog's tooth, still wrapped in finest silk, and began fervently to offer it prayers and prostrations. For hours and hours, days and days, she stayed at her shrine, locked in deep devotional prayer towards what she truly believed was the ancient tooth of Buddha himself.

After a while the son became concerned that his mother was becoming obsessed with what he knew to be nothing more than a poor ruse, so he went in to check on her. What he *saw amazed him. He found her totally mesmerized in deep meditative absorption, gazing at the silk wrap, which was now glowing and illuminated with rainbow-coloured light. By the extraordinary power of the woman's faith and devotional prayer, she had been granted the blessing of what she believed she was praying to and soon she became fully enlightened and attained rainbow body* upon her death.*

From the Tibetan Buddhist perspective, it's not just the object of your prayer that gives you the blessing, but the power of your prayer and strength of your devotion.

Throughout the Tibetan teachings on dream yoga we find advice to 'offer prayers that one may experience many dreams and that one may retain awareness in one's dreams'.[17] What you direct your prayers to is of course up to you, but I pray that you will give it a try.

Let Us Pray!

The word 'pray' found its way into Old English from the French *prier*, meaning 'to request', and although prayer is something far too personal to be taught as a method, here are a few suggestions on how you might like to word your requests for lucidity…

The great master Guru Rinpoche recommended reciting a dream yoga prayer to your spiritual teacher or a specific enlightened archetype using the following words: 'Bless me that I may recognize the dream state.'[18] This prayer, although short, carries the actual blessing of Guru Rinpoche, which is a very powerful blessing of course.

Another Buddhist dream yoga prayer comes from Lama Surya Das, who recommends reciting the following prayer while falling asleep:

---

* Rainbow body is a level of spiritual realization often accompanied by the phenomenon in which the physical body dissolves into coloured elemental light at the point of death, leaving nothing behind but the hair and fingernails.

'May I awaken within this dream and grasp the fact that I am
dreaming, so that all dreamlike beings may likewise awaken
from the nightmare of illusory suffering and confusion.'[19]

My favourite variation on this technique is to visualize an
embodiment of enlightenment (such Buddha or Jesus) in your
heart or throat area* as you are falling asleep, while at the same
time offering them the simple prayer: 'Bless me with your grace.
Let me dream with full lucidity for the benefit of all beings.'

Charlie says

'Nothing is more personal than prayer, so don't feel limited by the examples
of prayers made up by other people. Make up your own prayer if you want
to. I'm constantly making up new prayers for lucidity, which I recite to my
guru, Lama Yeshe Rinpoche, as I fall asleep. Some nights they're quite
informal, but as long as your motivation is genuine and your intent is
positive, the words don't have to be profound.'

MINDFULNESS OF DREAM & SLEEP MICRO-TECHNIQUES

'For the first time in my life I was looking forward to going to
sleep...'[20] CARLOS CASTANEDA

If we want to take these practices seriously then we have to train
in all aspects of sleep, not just the dream state. In the same way
that an athlete who is training for a specific discipline will train in
all areas of general fitness and athleticism, so we must train in all
areas of Mindfulness of Dream & Sleep, not just in the specific
discipline of lucid dreaming.

---

* Within Tibetan Buddhism, the throat chakra is associated strongly with lucid dreaming. Interestingly,
at a physical level, the area of the throat chakra is also where the brain stem originates. It is the brain
stem that stimulates REM dreaming.

In this chapter I have gathered together a variety of micro-techniques and personal tips based around embracing the practice and using every aspect of sleep as an aid on the path to lucidity. I've got dozens of my own Mindfulness of Dream & Sleep techniques, and because lucid dreaming is still a frontier land, you too can pioneer your own methods.

Preparing the Space

With so much of lucid dream induction being dependent upon intention, our actual preparation for sleep can be used as a lucid dreaming technique in itself.

The fact is that if we rush to bed, hurrying to get to sleep, or if we fall asleep on the couch with the TV blaring, we are unlikely to have lucid dreams. However, if we take some time before sleep to prepare the space of both our sleeping area and our mind, we will imbue our final minutes of wakefulness with the strong intention for lucidity. You wouldn't just 'stumble into' your yoga practice, would you? You'd lay out your yoga mat, make sure your phone was switched off, get a glass of water and prepare yourself mentally for your yoga session, right? You can do exactly the same thing for your dream yoga session. Plump up your pillows, make the bed if it is unmade, put on some relaxing music, dim the lights, do whatever you like to create an atmosphere of spiritual practice and ritual.

Lucid dreamers should enjoy preparing for each night's sleep and really look forward to going to bed, not only because they are excited at the prospect of lucid dreaming but also because they know that the more sacred they can make the process of going to sleep, the more likely they are to enter the sacred space of lucid dreams.

> **Charlie says**
>
> *'When I'm getting ready for a night of lucid dreaming, I sometimes feel as though I'm getting ready for a night of romance! I light the room with candles, offer incense over the bed, put on some beautiful music... I know it seems silly, but we're hardwired for ritual, so creating a ritual around going to bed can have a powerful effect.'*

Beat the Alarm

Have you ever forgotten to set your alarm clock but managed to wake yourself up at the right time anyway? If you have, you'll make a great lucid dreamer! Spontaneous awakening from intent is proof of the power of your prospective memory, which is the driving force behind the MILD technique and loads of other lucidity practices.

Don't just wait until you've forgotten to set your alarm clock, though – practise this technique at least once a week. Before you go to sleep, set the strong intention to wake up at a specific time in the morning without the use of an alarm clock. For beginners, I recommend setting an alarm clock for five minutes after you intend to wake yourself up, though, just in case you don't manage it the first time round!*

Have a Lie-in

You're going to love this one. Research has concluded that the probability of having a lucid dream in the last two hours of sleep is more than twice as great as in the previous six hours of sleep.**

---

* I once received an angry e-mail from a woman who blamed me and my 'stupid technique' for a written warning she had received from her boss for turning up late to work!

** If you already get seven or eight hours of sleep then you can take that up to 10 hours, but not more. Regularly having over 10 hours of sleep has been shown to be detrimental to health.

This means that you can almost double your chances of having a lucid dream by extending your sleep by an extra two hours! Still try to wake briefly at your normal time, though, rather than just sleeping straight through for the extra two hours, because then you get a chance to drop back into sleep while practising a lucidity technique.

Interestingly, from the perspective of Tibetan medicine, which sees our sleep cycle as broken up into stages of influence from each of the three humours of the body (bile, phlegm and subtle wind energy), the last two hours of the sleep cycle is when we experience 'the most balanced state of subtle wind energy' and thus the best time to engage in dream yoga practice.[21]

Change Position

There is a lot of different advice when it comes to the best sleeping position for inducing lucid dreams. Some schools of Tibetan Buddhism ask long-term retreatants to sleep upright in cross-legged meditation posture rather than lying down, so that their internal energy systems remain engaged throughout the night. Other schools say that we should 'sleep as the lion does', with our head facing north, lying on the right side of the body for men and the left side of the body for women.* I've tried all of these variations, plus quite a few more, and although many of them are very effective in inducing lucid dreams, I've also had many lucid dreams while sleeping on my front and back and somewhere in between, so although experimenting with different sleeping positions should be encouraged, don't feel that there is only one position in which you can have lucid dreams.

---

* This side-sleeping posture for dream practice has been found in a sculpture of the sleeping goddess of the Hypogeum in Malta dating from 3800–3600BCE. The Hypogeum was a space used for receiving prophetic healing dreams.

One tip that seems universal, though, is for heavy sleepers to have a slightly higher pillow, so that the head is raised. This seems to help maintain conscious awareness and prevent people from dropping off to sleep too quickly.

Get to Know How You Sleep

If we can become aware of how we sleep and the stages of our sleep cycle we can not only begin to timetable the most beneficial times to practise lucid dreaming techniques, but we can also gain a better understanding of how we sleep and dream. Every time that I wake up after a lucid dream I make a casual note of the time so that I can better understand when I have my greatest occurrence of lucid dreams and spontaneous wake-ups.

Charlie says

'It seems crazy that most of us know so little about an activity that we spend 30 years of our lives doing. We each sleep in a totally individual way, so get to know how you sleep and don't feel limited by what the scientists say about sleep stages – we all sleep in wonderfully abnormal ways and we must embrace that as part of this practice!'

Be Confident

After practical training, the next most important aspect of lucid dreaming and Mindfulness of Dream & Sleep is confidence in your own ability. Those of you who haven't had a lucid dream yet may think, *I don't have any ability!*, but remember that you used to lucid dream all the time when you were a child… And even if you haven't had a lucid dream yet as an adult, I'm sure that you've had some success in being aware of the hypnagogic and hypnopompic states or recalling your dreams. In fact, just by reading this book you are creating the causes and conditions that will lead to lucidity.

You can feel confident that lucidity will come soon as long as you keep practising. I've come across many people who have got lucid on their first night of practice and I've also come across people who have taken six months to have their first lucid dream. True confidence comes from the knowledge that you've put in the hard work, and confidence based on this knowledge is like the varnish on the treasure chest, sealing the grain of the wood, preserving and protecting its lustre. So, have confidence in yourself – you *are* a lucid dreamer!

As the full potential of lucid dreaming sinks in, some people find they get quite fanatical about the practice, and although we don't want to become too obsessed, we should allow ourselves to feel inspired. One of the best ways to get in touch with this inspiration is to really study lucid dreaming. Read books about lucid dreaming, watch films about lucid dreaming, read through your own lucid dreams to boost your confidence before bed and do whatever you can to imprint the importance of lucid dreaming into the foundation of your waking mind.

Charlie says

'Dreams occur in the mind, so they are directly influenced by your state of mind. If you go to sleep doubting your ability to have lucid dreams or not trusting in the techniques, then this will naturally hinder your ability to get lucid. Go to sleep in a confident state of mind and I'm confident that the techniques will work for you.'

Have Fun with the Practice

The Dalai Lama says that within the dream yoga teachings, an ancient method used by the monks was to buddy up and for one monk to watch the other sleep. When he saw the sleeper's eyes start to move rapidly, he would whisper in his ear, 'You are now dreaming. Recognize the dream state.'

Although you may not be a monk, you can still have lots of fun by trying out this technique for yourself. Try to rope in your partner or a friend to whisper lucidity cues into your ear as you sleep – it can be very effective, and a lot of fun, too. By letting our loved ones become part of our lucid dreaming practice, we might even inspire them to try it out as well.

Or not. Back in my early 20s, I tried using the voice recorder on my mobile phone as a lucid dream induction device by recording myself saying (in a rather pseudo-spiritual voice), 'Charlie, you are now dreammmming. What you are experiencing is just a dreammmm...' and then setting this voice recording as a 4 a.m. alarm in the hope that it would penetrate my dreaming consciousness as I slept. That night, however, my girlfriend stayed over unexpectedly, and I was awoken at 4 a.m. not by the alarm but by her mocking laughter as she heard my voice recording!

Charlie says

'If my teeny contribution to dream work could be anything, it would be to make it fun! Nobody ever said that spiritual practice should be boring and yet so many people present it in such a boring way. The great thing about these Mindfulness of Dream & Sleep techniques is that they are deeply transformative practices which also happen to be really fun to do.'

Read a Bedtime Story

Conventions of narrative and storytelling are things we learn not only from early childhood but throughout our adult lives from films, literature and performance. In our dream state, these narrative modes re-engage, and so people who consume a lot of film, theatre and literary narratives tend to have more complex dream narratives than those who consume fewer. On that basis, if we actively increase our intake of narrative, we may experience more vivid dreams.

Another great benefit of reading before bed is that it's been shown that reading activates the frontal cortex, which is the seat of analytical awareness and the part of the brain that recognizes we're dreaming.[22]

Recreational reading can also help reduce stress levels. This is the perfect preparation for both sleep and lucid dream practice, especially if you find that you have a bit of performance anxiety before bed. Scientists at the University of Sussex have found that reading for just six minutes cuts stress levels by up to 68 per cent[*] and that by reading you are 'actively engaging the imagination, as the words on the page stimulate your creativity and cause you to enter what is essentially an altered state of consciousness'.[23]

Buy the Hardware

There is a variety of lucid dreaming hardware available, ranging from computerized sleep masks that tell you when you're dreaming[**] to pillows with audio speakers inside them through which to play lucid dream induction audio tracks. There is also a range of brainwave-generating audio tracks that encourage our brain into certain states of consciousness, and countless lucid dreaming downloads and apps for computer or phone. I've tried loads of these, with varying degrees of success, but as long as they are seen as aids to our training (like stabilizers on a bicycle) and not replacements, they might prove quite helpful.

---

[*] Sixty-eight per cent reduction in stress within six minutes? There's no known anti-stress medicine on the market that can claim those results. Amazing!

[**] The mask contains sensors that recognize REM and send out a flash of red light bright enough to penetrate our eyelids, but not bright enough to wake us up, so that it enters our dream and cues lucidity.

Be mindful, though, that getting attached to a certain brainwave soundscape playing as you fall asleep or to wearing a computerized sleep mask can soon become an obstacle to your practice. As the dream yogi Tenzin Rinpoche once told me, 'You won't have your fancy sleep mask when you enter the *bardo!*'[24]

There are also certain foodstuffs that contain chemicals beneficial to sleeping* as well as B-vitamin supplements – which may lead to more vivid dreams – and even anti-Alzheimer's drugs, which offer easy lucidity.** Be careful about getting into the habit of popping a pill before a lucid dreaming session, though. The way I look at it is like this: if somebody produced a pill for meditation, would I take it? Definitely not – meditation practice is called practice because it's exactly that – and we shouldn't try and usurp it with chemicals.

Improve your Balance

It seems that if we can keep our physical balance in real life, we will be better equipped to keep our mental balance in the lucid dream. Studies have shown that people who have good spatial skills and physical body balance seem to have a natural propensity for lucid dreaming.*** The reason behind these findings is that an important component of both physical balance and lucid dreaming is the vestibular system of balance (a kind of spirit level in the inner ear), which is linked to the production of eye

---

* Foods such as raw (unpasteurized) milk and cheese contain amino acids that have been proven to stimulate the production of melatonin, a vital neurotransmitter for sleeping and dreaming. So having a glass of milk before bed may be good advice.

** I am of course talking about Galantamine, a memory-enhancing drug that, if taken in the early hours of the morning, can often lead to lucidity. I do not recommend it, but I will save my rant for Chapter 9.

*** A friend from South Africa actually started tightrope walking in view of this. Perhaps it was just coincidence, but that friend became an outstanding lucid dreamer and now actually co-facilitates courses with me.

movements during REM sleep. Those with a more developed vestibular system, such as martial artists, dancers and tightrope walkers, seem to have the potential for extended REM periods and more lucid dreams.

So what about those of us who are not one of the above? Try balancing on one leg for five minutes a day, learn a martial art, take up ballroom dancing or do whatever you can to improve your physical balance.

Be Enthusiastic

The American philosopher Ralph Waldo Emerson said, 'Enthusiasm is the mother of effort, and without it nothing great was ever achieved.' If you want to learn how to lucid dream regularly, then lucid dreaming has to be something you're enthusiastic about. Lama Zangmo, the female Lama who runs the Buddhist centre where I live, says that the most important aspect of lucid dream training is enthusiasm. She told me that 'the main thing is to have a very strong intention. You have to be fired up for it, you have to really want to do it!'[25] Sometimes I feel a real sense of excitement before I go to bed because I've prepared and motivated myself so much – doing reality checks throughout the day, reading about lucid dreaming before bed, setting multiple alarms to go off throughout the night, etc. – that the act of falling asleep is like going on stage to perform.

This is an extreme example, but it exemplifies just how enthusiastic you can become about lucid dreaming, and perhaps even how enthusiastic you need to become if you really want to master it.

Look on the Bright Side

New lucid dreamers may find that they become quite fixated and inflexible regarding their 'precious sleep' as they plan out every minute of sleep and curse anything that disrupts it. But relax, because it seems that there is a bright side to almost all sleep disruptions.

Anything that mildly disrupts our sleeping patterns leads to our consciousness spending more time in the lighter levels of sleep, which is where lucid dreams occur most readily. Having to change our sleeping area by sleeping on hotel beds, planes, trains or friends' sofas is often seen as an irritation to our practice but actually it is very conducive to lucid dreaming because it can lead to changes in our sleeping pattern and a heightened state of awareness as we sleep.

Interruptions to our sleep cycle should also be welcomed, because, as we know, being woken several times during the night offers us several opportunities to become lucid. Suddenly, drunk flatmates, noisy neighbours and barking dogs can be embraced on the path! So, whatever your night-time disturbances, try to look on the bright side.

Charlie says

'I am forever thankful for the rumblings of my dad's snoring, which would plough through the walls of my bedroom when I was learning how to lucid dream. I used to wake up, acknowledge the sound of the snoring and then fall asleep again, consciously using the sound to anchor my awareness. It was a real blessing. I don't think my mum saw it that way, though.'

Be Kind

Our mind's energy is affected by everything we do, think and say, so if we spend our waking hours engaged in negative, harmful or unkind activities, this will naturally lead to the negative disturbance of our mindstream during our dreaming hours, too, making the mindful awareness needed to lucid dream unlikely.

So I propose that as part of our lucid dreaming training we

should actively seek to be kind to ourselves and to others during everyday life. This will not only create beneficial mind energy while we are being kind, but will also create the perfect karmic conditions in which to practise lucid dreaming that night.

Charlie says

'Every time you have a lucid dream, look back on the day preceding it and try and find patterns to your behaviour that might boost your lucidity. A few years back, when I was still working in the hip-hop scene, I started to find that I kept having spontaneous lucid dreams the night after I'd been teaching kids rapping and poetry. For me it seems that prolonged creative right-brain engagement fills my lucidity tank to the brim. What fills up your lucidity tank?'

So, you now have a fully stocked toolbox of lucidity techniques! Whether you actually use the tools and what you choose to build with them is up to you, but I can assure you that you now have everything you need to become a fully certified lucid dream handyman, or woman.

There is a Zen Buddhist teaching that says spiritual practice is like eating food. You can't gain the nourishment of food just from reading about it, talking about it or learning about the ingredients – you actually have to eat it. It's exactly the same with lucid dreaming. So let's go to sleep and eat.

'I'm Lucid – What Now?'

*'We may judge of your natural character by what
you do in your dreams.'*
RALPH WALDO EMERSON

I often get e-mails from new lucid dreamers saying that they 'finally got lucid' but then didn't know what to do once they were! Fully lucid dreams can be quite elusive when we first start out on the path, so it's a good idea to spend some time working out what we want to do once we have one. It's much better to give this question some thought in the waking state than trying to think about it once we're in the lucid dream. In fact, planning what we want to do in our lucid dream is a very powerful induction method, too.*

When we find ourselves fully lucid within the amazingly realistic three-dimensional dreamscape, the question of what to do becomes limited only by our imagination and the strength of our friendship with our unconscious mind. For those of you interested in the practice of dream yoga, this is really where the path starts

---

* The lack of left-brain activation in the first few seconds of lucidity can make logical reasoning tasks quite hard to engage, so I advise you to do your lucid dream planning in the waking state rather than doing it ad hoc within the dream.

in earnest. As B. Alan Wallace says, you should use whatever methods you can to become lucid, because once you are, 'that is the basis for whatever dream yoga activities you choose to enact'.[1]

Our level of volitional influence over our lucid dreams will increase with practice, and with sustained training we can get to a level where we can literally do anything our unconscious allows, without any constraints from the laws of physics. Certain activities may *seem* more difficult to engage in than others, but this is due to the limits of our expectations rather than the limits of the dream. The dream is limitless.

When engaging intentional action in the lucid dream, the most important thing to remember is that *manifestation follows thought* or, as the Buddha said, 'With our thoughts we make the world.' Robert Waggoner comments, 'The dream space largely mirrors your ideas, expectations and beliefs about it. By changing your expectations and beliefs, you change the dream space.'[2]

So how does it actually work? To engage in any lucid dream activity, affirm your intent once you become lucid, either mentally or out loud, and then engage in your chosen activity with full confidence, holding in mind at all times the fact that you are dreaming.* It may sound simplistic, but when you're operating in a world of mental constructs, it's your thoughts, words and expectations that dictate what happens. So, you have to be mindful of your mind throughout the process.

Of course, there are countless activities you can get up to in your dream world, and if you already have some ideas cooking then feel free to skip ahead, but here are my personal 'top ten' lucid dream activities, which I can say for sure can be of both psychological and spiritual benefit and also a whole lot of fun. Here they are in ascending order...

---

* Stating your intent mentally is fine of course, but I recommend that beginners state their intent out loud, because that seems to help concretize the intent in a clearer and more precise way.

LUCIDITY IN ACTION TOP TEN
Number 10: Life Rehearsal

Coming in at number ten is using the lucid dream for rehearsing new mental habits and alternative ways of interacting with the world.

In the lucid dream you can work on aspects of your own psychology in a totally safe virtual reality of your own creation. If you are a very shy person, you can use a lucid dream to practise being more outgoing. If you are a very proud person, you can use a lucid dream to practise acting more humbly. Whatever change you want to make in the waking state can be started in the safety of a lucid dream – a laboratory of change in which mistakes can be made and new perspectives explored without fear of failure.

The lucid dream state can also be a wonderful training ground for motor-skill recapitulation and for creating blueprints for physical action that will stay activated in the waking state. So within the dream we can spend time rehearsing physical activities like sport, yoga or even physical rehabilitation, which will (as we learned in Chapter 4) lead to a neurological pathway being grooved into the plasticity of our brain that will make these activities easier to perform in the waking state.

Let's Do It!

Once lucid, simply engage in the action or habit that you wish to practise, just as you would when awake but free from the waking state's limitations.

You can visualize yourself in the space where you would normally perform this action, but it's not essential. It's more important just to do it – and to be mindful of the feelings and sensations that occur while you're engaging in it.

These feelings and sensations will reappear like real-life memories when you next perform the action in the waking state.

Charlie says

'Dancing in public is a nightmare for many people. Personally, after ten years of working with breakdancers, I found that dancing for me was tied up with machismo and with "dancing well". When I took up expressive dance forms like 5 Rhythms and Movement Medicine, I decided to try to move beyond this old habit. The lucid dream state was the perfect place to have a quick rehearsal for this and it changed the way I danced forever!'
(For a full description of this dream, see Dream 1, page 241.)

Number 9: See the Bigger Picture

An entire menu for a three-day residential retreat, much of this book and part of a TED talk are just three of the bigger-picture creative endeavours that I engaged within the lucid dream state. The pioneer of quantum consciousness, Professor Amit Goswami, believes, 'If one can tune oneself to the creative characteristics of the dream state, then we can use the dream state to develop these creative qualities within ourselves.'[3]

The natural dominance of the right brain in the dream state is what makes it such a great place to see the bigger picture. Neurologists tell us the right hemisphere is, 'by its design, spontaneous and imaginative... [a place in which] our artistic juices flow freely without inhibition or judgement'.[4] Often, however, our lack of awareness in our dreams means that we miss out on the potential our right hemisphere offers. Once we bring lucid left-brain cognizance into a dream, though, we are in direct communication with the right hemisphere and able to benefit from the insights it offers – and from its ability to see the bigger picture.

This makes the lucid dream state the perfect place for reflecting on life choices and asking for advice from the unconscious mind.

Let's Do It!

Once you become lucid, state out loud your creative task or 'bigger-picture' question such as 'How can I finish my poem?' or 'What career path should I take?'

Be aware of any changes to the dreamscape or any newly formed dream characters who might hold the answer to your question, and remember, the answer may not come in the form you would expect.

Charlie says

'A few years back I was really doubting whether I was qualified to teach dream work as a career. I felt too young and inexperienced to have much to offer. After a few weeks of wrestling with this, I had a lucid dream in which I asked for some advice. My dreaming mind encouraged me to follow my dreams. It was one of the most important lucid dreams of my life.' (For a full description of this dream, see Dream 2, page 242.)

Number 8: Interact with Internal Archetypes

From Will Smith to the Dalai Lama, deceased grandmothers to Bollywood film stars, conjuring up that special someone in a lucid dream seems to be a goal for many people. But using the lucid dream to meet internal psychological archetypes rather than Will Smith is much more beneficial in my opinion.

Once we are dreaming, we can also ask to meet aspects of our own psychology in personified form. We can have a conversation with our higher self, meet our subconscious or even talk to our inner child.

Let's Do It! 🦋🦋

Once you're lucid, simply call out your request, for example: 'I want to meet my inner child! Inner child, come to me!' and then either simply wait for them to appear or actively engage in a search for them.

Carefully scan your surroundings once you have made your request because they may appear in a form that you did not expect.

Once they appear, engage them in conversation. Ask them what they represent or simply embrace them with love and kindness.

Charlie says 💬

'I will never forget the first time I intentionally met a psychological archetype. It changed my life forever. It was the dream in which I met the personification of my subconscious mind!' (For a full description of this dream, see Dream 3, page 244.)

Number 7: Ask 'Big Questions'

In at number seven is using the lucid dream to ask big questions such as: What is the nature of reality? Is the future already written? Is there a God? These are the kind of big questions that humankind has been investigating since time began. A great way to further these investigations is to ask these questions in the lucid dream state.

Your big question might be something personally significant or globally significant, but whatever it is, make sure that you really want to hear the answer that your dreaming mind will offer.

The enlightened knowledge that we all possess can often seem quite inaccessible in the waking state, but through lucid dreaming we can gain access to it much more easily, and perhaps even to the collective wisdom beyond the dream.

Let's Do It! 🦋

Take a few moments before bed to affirm your intent. Let your unconscious know that you are looking to it for insight and guidance.

In your next lucid dream, simply state your question out loud to the dreaming mind – call it out to the sky or an open space rather than address it to a specific dream character.*

The reply you get may be as obvious as an immediate audible response or as subtle as a symbolic change to the dreamscape, so make sure that once you have raised your question you keep your senses engaged, ready to receive your answer in whatever form it may come.

There is also a self-hypnosis technique in which you imagine a TV screen and then address questions to it, imagining it to be your subconscious. The answer to your questions is then displayed on the screen in the form of words or an image.[5] This is a great technique to use within a lucid dream, but use whatever form works best for you.

Charlie says

'The first time I tried this dream plan I decided to aim high. I became lucid and yelled out to the dream, "What is the essence of all knowledge?" The answer I received revealed both the humour and the wisdom of the unconscious mind. It's amazing the answers you can get if you only take the time to ask!' (For a full description of this dream, see Dream 4, page 245.)

---

* If you pose your question to a specific dream character, the answer you get may be tainted by your unconscious assumptions of that particular dream character, so it is far better to pose your question to the dreaming mind itself.

Number 6: Walk through Walls

When I was trying to get my head round the concept of emptiness with Rob Nairn one day, he told me, 'It's only doubt that stops us walking through walls.'[6] I agreed with him, because I once had a lucid dream in which I got stuck halfway through a wall, and I put this down to a moment of doubt. He looked at me, smiled and said, 'I wasn't talking about lucid dreams, I was talking about real life.'

In both dream and waking reality, nothing is fixed; everything contains infinite possibility and exists in a state of dreamlike interdependence and quantum potentiality. Professor of quantum physics Lenny Susskind says, 'Quantum mechanics says that I can pass through that wall. How often will it happen? Very rarely, but wait long enough and it will happen.'[7] In a lucid dream we don't have to wait that long.

Tibetan dream yoga teachings advise the dreamer to explore the infinite potentiality of the dream by 'trying to go through walls'.[8] This is a way not only to gain ultimate insight into the illusory nature of dream projections but also to systematically train the mind to break through the habit of viewing solid things as impenetrable. The esteemed dream yogi Namkai Norbu Rinpoche says that if we can use the lucid dream state to 'pass through seemingly solid walls, this is a very favourable experience for overcoming the attachments of daily life because we experience directly the insubstantiality and unreality of all things'.[9]

. . . .

Let's Do It! 🦋

Once lucid within the dream, find a solid surface or wall. Remind yourself that this hard surface is actually a mental construct with no solidity at all and simply pass your hand through it or into it.*

---

* It's common to feel some physical resistance while passing through an object. This is the mind trying to maintain the illusion of solidity that it habitually engages. Just remind yourself: this is the stuff that dreams are made of.

Then once you feel brave enough, try walking or running through a wall. Some people like to wade into the wall very slowly, experiencing fully the sensations of solidity or liquidity, while others like to run full pelt into the wall! There is no 'best practice' as far as this is concerned.

False awakenings are a common occurrence with this technique, so be sure to do a reality check straight afterwards.

Charlie says

'Every time we walk through a wall in a lucid dream we are creating a new habit, a new neural pathway in our brain. This new pathway says, "That which seems solid is not always so." Cultivation of such a revolutionary new habit affects our waking life in that we come to see the solidity of emotions, prejudices and fears as similarly unsolid.' (For a full description of this technique, see Dream 5, page 246.)

Number 5: Heal

Hitting our chart at number five is one of my all-time favourite applications of lucid dreaming: healing. To engage this technique, all you require is some sort of physical or mental ailment that you would like to heal.

I have healed everything from mental addictions to ear infections through this method, so it doesn't matter what the ailment is, only that you have the strong belief that you can heal it through lucid dreaming.

'But that's just the placebo effect!' the cynics cry. That's right, but as the famously sceptical Dr Ben Goldacre says, 'The proof of the placebo effect is an outrageous and ridiculous finding, but it's true. It's all about our beliefs and expectations.'[10] As we know, the lucid dream state is influenced in large part by our expectations, which is why it is the perfect place to engage the placebo effect.

Buddhist scholar B. Alan Wallace says, 'It should be called the mind effect, not the placebo effect! It's all about the mind affecting the body.'[11] The lucid dream is a state of pure mind and so the 'mind effect' works with maximum efficacy when engaged within it.

Let's Do It! 🦋🦋

Once lucid, state out loud your healing intent, for example 'I am free of any and all non-beneficial disease' or 'I am healed, all is well,' while directing healing intent to the area of disease or discomfort.

If the ailment has a physical component, then place your hands on the affected area within the dream and intend that healing light flows from your hands into the area that needs healing.

To engage healing for another person you either call up a visualized projection of them within the lucid dream and apply hands-on healing or simply direct statements of healing intent towards them.

> **Charlie says**
>
> *'I had heard of loads of people healing themselves from physical ailments through lucid dreaming, but I had never experienced it first hand. That was until I contracted a rather nasty ear infection from surfing and proceeded to heal it in a lucid dream.'* (For a full description of this dream, see Dream 6, page 248.)

Number 4: Explore the Emptiness of the Dream

Through lucid dreaming we can experience the empty nature of the dream by simply exploring the dreamscape in the knowledge that it is a mental fabrication. This is quite an experience to have.

Back in Chapter 4 we explored how the Buddhist term 'emptiness' actually meant pure potentiality and how because something was empty of inherent existence it could contain infinite possibility. In the lucid dream state we can experience emptiness directly because we can see how everything that seems real and solid is just a projection of our own mind, totally impermanent and brimming with infinite manifestations.

Exploring the empty nature of the dream is an instruction from the Tibetan dream yoga teachings, which advise the lucid dreamer to explore the seemingly solid appearance of the illusory dreamscape as a way of appreciating the dreamlike nature of waking reality.

These same Tibetan teachings also actively encourage us to transform the dreamscape we are exploring: 'if the dream be of minute objects, transform them into large objects' and 'if the dream be of a single thing, transform it into many things'.[12]

This kind of direct manipulation of the dreamscape may sound a bit like domination and control, but if it is engaged in with the motivation of exploring the dreamscape and, through that, exploring emptiness, then I'm sure the unconscious won't mind.

Let's Do It!

Once lucid, simply walk or fly around the dreamscape and explore it, resolute in the knowledge that everything you're experiencing is an elaborately detailed mental construct.

Keep reminding yourself that everything is made of mind as you touch things, smell things, see if things are solid or energetic, feel the different textures of the ground or the buildings or the water. Eating something, touching the hair on your head and feeling the beating heart of your dream body are personal recommendations of mine.

Be sure to keep in mind the understanding that what you are experiencing is a dream, because sometimes too much engagement in a dreamscape that looks very real can make you forget this.

Once you feel comfortable with exploring, try to transform certain elements of the dreamscape. Maybe make an object grow larger or smaller. This will help you to explore the plasticity of both the dream and your own mind. As you do so, always maintain an attitude of respect for the dream, of course.

Charlie says

'To explore the lucid dream world is to explore the true nature of reality. To enter into the awareness that everything in the dream is created by the mind is to enter into a relationship with quantum creativity and with emptiness. Emptiness is a big concept to understand fully, but in the lucid dream we can at least begin to explore it.' (For a full description of this technique, see Dream 7, page 249.)

Number 3: Receive Teachings

Rolling in at number 3 is receiving teachings and advice within the lucid dream. As I mentioned in Part I, I believe that lucid dreams can be the medium through which we can receive teachings from our own innate wisdom essence, sometimes called our Buddha nature or higher self. But perhaps we can receive teachings from sources outside ourselves, too?

The dream yoga teachings state that lucid dreams can be an excellent medium through which to receive spiritual teachings from the mindstream of enlightened masters, and some lamas even advise us to actively seek out such teachings by getting lucid and going to other realms of existence 'to study and see the teachers who live in these holy places'.[13]

Let's Do It! 🦋🦋

Sometimes teachings will come to us without a request being made at all. To receive these teachings, the most important thing is to maintain a non-preferential openness to whatever our innate wisdom mind presents us with, because often the teachings will come to us in a way that we don't expect.

Alternatively, we can ask for teachings directly. I recommend stating your intent out loud to the dream, saying something like 'Higher self, teach me how I can be of benefit!' or 'Show me how to realize my full potential!' or 'Inner guru, come to me!'

If you have a link to a spiritual teacher, you can also call out for them to offer you teachings. If they arrive and start teaching you, remember they may be just a mental projection or an actual aspect of that teacher. Only you can know for sure.

Charlie says

'Sometimes the teachings that I've received in a lucid dream have been so precise and so seemingly unknown to me that I've found myself opening to the possibility that they have been sourced from something outside my own personal mindstream. We can never know for sure, but if the teachings we receive are based on kindness and compassion then maybe it doesn't matter where they are from anyway.' (For a full description of a teaching lucid dream, see Dream 8, page 250, and Dream 18, page 263.)

Number 2: Integrate the Shadow

Almost at the top of the chart, we find lucid dream shadow integration. As mentioned in Part I, the shadow is a Jungian concept used to describe the parts of the unconscious mind that are made up of all the undesirable aspects of our psyche that we have rejected, disowned and denied. Nevertheless, these are aspects of ourselves that we need not fear.

The shadow is often misinterpreted as some sort of evil or demonic presence that is both separate from us and harmful to us, leading us to waste the valuable learning process it offers us by investing our energy in ways to defeat it. The truth is that the shadow is neither external nor harmful. It is our 'dark side', but, as Jung commented, 'In spite of its function as a reservoir for human darkness – or perhaps because of this – the shadow is the seat of all creativity.'[14] It is part of us and until we accept that its darkness doesn't come from an external 'evil' but from a wellspring of internal creative energy, we will never be able to be a fully integrated human being.

The main benefit of shadow integration in both the waking world and the dream world is the psychotherapeutic one of the assimilation of rejected shadow aspects into the wholeness of the Self, leading to what Jung termed 'individuation' or full psychological completeness.

In lucid dreams a shadow aspect may take on personified form as obviously as a nightmarish monster rampaging towards us, or as subtly as a dream character who is just particularly repellent. But whatever form it takes, rather than running from it, fighting it or arguing with it, we should remain lucid, fearless and patient as we embrace it with the compassionate realization that it is merely a mental construct of our own shadow, which we now have the valuable opportunity to integrate.

Vajrayana Buddhism is all about shadow integration and there is a great metaphor used to describe it: the peacock that eats the poison. It's believed that the source of the peacock's beautiful plumage is the poisonous plants that it eats, and that it is the alchemical transmutation of this poison that gives it the colours of its plume. The teachings tell us that we too can 'transform the poisons of ignorance, attachment and aversion into the medicine of wisdom and compassion'[15] and so with that in mind, we can be confident that shadow integration will allow us to transform negative emotions into enlightened potential.

Compared to the content of non-lucid dreams, research has shown that lucid dreams tend to be more emotionally positive experiences, perhaps because the parts of the brain that mediate fear and other emotions, as well as those that control hallucinatory perception, aren't as dominant as they are in non-lucid dreams. This is because our knowledge that what we are experiencing is 'just a dream' regulates our emotions.

Lucid dreams may be overwhelmingly positive experiences leading to feelings of great joy and accomplishment at having finally recognized the illusion that has duped us for so long. However, it's not all plain sailing, because some people find that disturbing shadow aspects appear *more* frequently in lucid dreams than in non-lucid ones. The reason for this, I believe, may be due to another Jungian theory called 'compensation'. Jung described compensation as 'an inherent self-regulation in the psychic apparatus'[16] that aims for harmonious balance within the psyche of both the accepted aspects of ourselves and the rejected aspects, the dark with the light. Lucid dreams in which we just focus on fluffy bunnies and blue skies may disrupt this balance and call forth something a little darker.

This phenomenon should therefore be seen as a great opportunity, offering us lots of chances to embrace the shadow aspects we encounter in the dream as part of ourselves and to face them fearlessly, understanding completely, as Shakespeare did, that this 'thing of darkness I acknowledge as mine'.[17]

Let's Do It!

The fundamental way to practise shadow integration in lucid dreams is that whenever we encounter a frightening, perverted, violent or distasteful dream character or dream scenario, we should actively embrace it with love, rather than either running away or rejecting it through violence.[*]

Actively embracing it might mean something as literal as hugging it or as subtle as turning and facing it with acceptance and courage. It's about doing the opposite of what we usually do when we meet our shadow, which is to turn away from it.

Deepak Chopra says, 'If you want authentic peace of mind, creativity and joy, then you have to understand your shadow, and to celebrate it.'[18] So don't try and wake yourself up when you meet your shadow; instead try and stay with it, fearless in the knowledge that it is part of you, a mental projection of aspects of your own psyche.

If you want to take this technique one step further then you might like to try intentionally calling out for your shadow in the lucid dream. This is one of the most deeply healing lucid dream practices in existence, but it comes with a caveat... If you call out 'Shadow, come to me!' in a lucid dream, you'd better be ready for it, because you've just opened the floodgates and called forth the totality of your darkness. Although this technique is absolutely safe (and in fact the shadow will only present you with what you are ready for), I advise that you try it only when you are feeling very grounded.

---

* Shadow integration and fearlessness in dreams may naturally start to manifest in our waking world, too. We begin to see aspects of our own negative projections that we can integrate, just as we have trained to do in the dream.

If you do manage to meet your shadow face to face, I recommend that you give it a hug and show it love. Doing so may be the single most important thing you will ever do.

Charlie says

'Shadow integration is one of the most powerful psychological healing techniques available to the lucid dreamer. In just one lucid dream we can make strides towards healing and integration that might have taken years in the waking state. We can directly converse with personified shadow aspects and even dissolve them into our own dream body as a symbol of full integration.' (For a full description of this practice, see Dream 9, page 251, and for another great shadow integration dream, see Dream 14, page 257.)

Number 1: Do Spiritual Practice

And at number one in my top ten chart we have spiritual practice in the lucid dream! This can be a truly powerful experience and it's my all-time favourite thing to do once lucid.

During the waking state our spiritual practice is often hindered by the limitations of our physical body and energetic flow, but within the lucid dream state we are unhindered by these and can consequently reach levels of meditation which far surpass our waking practice.

The fruition of certain Tantric Buddhist practices of deity self-visualization is the actual manifestation of yourself as the deity or archetype you are visualizing. This can take decades of intense practice to manifest in the waking state (if at all), but in the lucid dream state we can manifest in the form of the deity much more easily. This is very beneficial for our spiritual practice because it leaves an energetic imprint in our waking mindstream.

If taking on the form of a buddha seems a bit too far out, even simply saying a few mantras or prayers within a lucid dream or meditating for a few seconds has immense energetic benefits, because, as we learned earlier, just one moment of spiritual practice in the lucid dream state is worth a one-week meditation retreat in the waking state! Now, *that's* time management!

Let's Do It!

Once you are lucid, engage in your spiritual practice. Whether it is sitting meditation, mantra recitation or saying prayers of healing, just carry out the practice exactly the same way as you would while in the waking state.

Remember, though, in the lucid dream you don't need a meditation cushion or prayer beads or a temple in order to do your spiritual practice, so wherever you are when you become lucid, just get straight into it.

Meditation in lucid dreams can often lead to incredibly strong sensations and experiences, so the most important thing is to stay grounded in the awareness that it is all a fabrication of the mind.

Charlie says

'Spiritual practice is my favourite activity to engage within a lucid dream. I've had loads of experiences of meditating in the lucid dream state, but one of the most profound experiences I've had was actually when I tried it for the first time. I was only 19 and I didn't really know what I was doing. It totally blew my mind and when I woke up I felt as if a curtain had been lifted.' (For a full description of this experience, see Dream 10, page 252.)

LUCID DREAM PLANNING

So, it seems that in lucid dreams we can do virtually anything we want to, right? This, of course, is not necessarily a beneficial thing and it should be noted that the lucid dream state can easily be used to indulge in non-beneficial actions.* Lama Surya Das says that 'lucid dreaming can easily be misused to perpetuate the problems we experience in our waking lives'[19] and I wholeheartedly agree. So it's best to plan ahead.

Lucid dream planning can also be a lucid dream induction technique in itself. It works in a similar way to dream incubation in that when we set a strong intention for our next lucid dream, we not only attract the causes and conditions needed to make that lucid dream manifest but we also create an expectation of becoming lucid.

Let's Plan!

Lucid dream plans can be created either in writing or in your head, but if you are just beginning, I would recommend that you write them out, so that you have a record of your progress for future reference.**

Using a section of your dream diary, draft some ideas of what you would like to do in your next lucid dream. What question would you like to ask? What activity would you like to engage in? What part of your psyche would you like to interact with?

Once you have decided what you want to do, begin to formulate your dream plan. A dream plan can be as simple as 'Tonight, when I lucid dream I want to meet my shadow and engage the parts of my psyche that I have repressed.' Your dream plan can be a long

---

* I think of the lucid dream state as a blank canvas within the art studio of the unconscious mind, so be mindful of what you paint.

** I always have at least three dream plans on the go so that I'm never left lost for inspiration once I'm lucid. Always have several plans on the back burner, too.

and detailed as you like, but I recommend that you keep it short and sharp.

Once you have formulated your dream plan, edit it, removing any unnecessary words or superfluous details. This will not only make it easier to remember but it will help to highlight its essence.

Once you are happy that your plan is complete, the next step is to create a *sangkalpa*,* or statement of intent. This should be a pithy statement that sums up the essence of your dream plan.

If your dream plan is to meet your shadow and engage the parts of your psyche that you have repressed, for example, then your *sangkalpa* to be stated out loud might be 'Shadow now!'– a much more pithy version of the quite wordy dream plan. If your dream plan is to walk through a wall, your *sangkalpa* might be just to remind yourself that 'This wall is an illusion' as you approach the wall.

Now commit the plan and *sangkalpa* to memory. As you fall asleep that night, remind yourself of your dream plan and engage your favourite lucid dream induction method.

The final step occurs when you next find yourself in a lucid dream. Once you get lucid, recall your dream plan, recite your *sangkalpa* out loud and carry out your chosen activity.

Charlie says

'Sometimes, once you get lucid you find that your dream plan is already being put into action by your unconscious mind. I think that when this happens it's a sign that your unconscious is totally on board with that dream plan and has been waiting for you to arrive so that it can get the show on the road!'

---

* *Sangkalpa* is a Sanskrit word meaning 'will', 'purpose' or 'determination'.

MAINTAINING LUCIDITY

Have you ever been to the circus and looked up at the tightrope walker balancing on the high wire, unfazed by the huge drop either side? Maintaining lucidity is just the same in that it's about balance. On one side of the lucidity tightrope there is non-lucid dreaming and on the other side there is the waking state. Just as a novice tightrope walker might only be able to take a few steps at first and stay on the wire for just a few seconds, so a novice lucid dreamer might only be lucid for a few brief moments. But with sustained practice we will eventually be balanced up on the wire for as long as we wish – maybe even doing backflips along it!

For many beginners, the difficulty is not so much getting on the lucidity spectrum as staying there. The 'Aha!' moment of lucid awareness is often followed by a rush of adrenaline which can be so strong that we lose our balance and fall off the tightrope into the waking state. The first few realizations of 'I'm lucid! I'm actually lucid!' can be so exhilarating that we can find ourselves awake in our bed, still buzzing with excitement, before we have actually had time to engage in any lucid exploration.

On the other hand, we can fall the other way, into non-lucid dreaming. This is usually caused by becoming distracted and forgetting that we're dreaming. Our attention is often diverted by some bizarre or attractive element of the dreamscape. This is like the tightrope walker who spots a waving child in the audience below and, in that split-second of distraction, slips and falls.

The Tibetan masters advise us that we should 'try and extend the periods of lucidity for longer and longer',[20] so we should really try and keep our balance on the lucidity tightrope for as long as possible. Don't forget, the lucid dream state is a more refined level of consciousness, so every second of lucidity is beneficial and healing for our mind.

There are loads of techniques for maintaining lucidity, but here are a few of my favourites, which I've found can maintain lucid awareness for extended periods of time. In fact, using these techniques I have even been able to maintain lucidity throughout an entire 60-minute REM period.*

'Keep Calm and Carry On!'

Older readers may remember the famous slogan of the British Home Office that encouraged Londoners to 'Keep calm and carry on' during the bombing raids of the Second World War. We need to 'keep calm and carry on dreaming' in order to avoid the panic of waking up when the bombs of distraction start falling.

The first part of this technique is simply to apply whatever we would do to keep calm in the waking state to the lucid dream state. Once we realize that we're lucid, we might feel the tightrope start to wobble a bit, but if we actively try to keep calm and mentally stable, we should be able to regain our balance. For me, this usually means saying to myself, 'OK, Charlie, keep calm. Breathe. It's all a dream. Keep calm.'

The second part of the technique is to 'carry on', because the lucid dream likes movement and if we stay too still or prevaricate about what we want to do, we may find that the lucidity begins to slip.

Lucidity Boost

If we feel the sense of lucid awareness start to fade, we can enhance our lucidity by stating out loud within the dream, 'Lucidity boost!' or 'Amplify lucidity!', which will lead to an increase in lucid awareness as well as a sharpening of detail in the dreamscape.

---

* As we learned before, estimation of time in the lucid dream state is the same as in the waking state. So if it feels as though you've been lucid for 10 minutes, you probably have been.

I know this sounds crazy, but it seems that while we are lucid dreaming, an aspect of our mind sometimes called the 'conscious-unconscious' is aware of what we are doing and so can increase lucid awareness upon command. The command is at its most impressive just at the point at which the lucid awareness is fading, but it can also be used right at the start of the lucid dream as a way of increasing clarity and mental focus.

Give and Take

If you want to maintain lucidity for extended periods of time you need to maintain a delicate balance between objective detachment and subjective participation. You have to be aware of the dream but also totally aware that it is a mental projection that you are dreaming into existence. Too much detachment from the dream and you may fall into a semi-lucid state or simply wake up. Too much over-engagement in the dream and you may slip into the all-encompassing self-identification that characterizes non-lucid dreams. Active participation is vital to engage the lucid potential of the dream and to maintain the conscious understanding that 'because I am dreaming this dream, I can influence it', but detachment is also needed in order to maintain objective awareness and the conscious understanding that 'this is all just a dream and I am dreaming it'. On the tightrope of lucidity, balance is key!

Arm Rubbing and Hand Checking

This technique isn't hard to explain: if your lucidity starts to slip, begin rubbing the arms of your dream body and/or perform hand reality checks. This is not only a great way to remind yourself that you are still dreaming (due to the hand reality checks) but it's also a great way to bring your attention back to the somatic awareness of your body.

Your body is likely to be one of the few constants in the lucid dream – while the dreamscape may be morphing around you, your body will probably remain unchanged. By bringing your awareness back to your body, you bring your mind back into check.

Spinning

This is a classic LaBergian technique used to maintain lucidity and simply consists of spinning around in your lucid dream. It works by harnessing the vestibular system of balance, which is found in the inner ear and not only helps to integrate information about bodily movement into the neurological system (which creates our visual experience of the world) but is also linked to the rapid eye movements of REM sleep.

It seems that the act of spinning around in a lucid dream tricks the mind into activating the vestibular system just as it would if we were spinning while awake, and this helps to maintain REM sleep and thus the stability of the dream.

Let's Do It!

As the visual dreamscape in your lucid dream begins to break up or fade, stretch out your arms* and spin around like a whirling dervish. As you do this, the dreamscape will often blur into a haze of motion or fade to black.

While you are spinning, hold the intention 'The next thing I see will be the reformed dreamscape' or 'I am spinning in order to maintain lucidity.'

After you have spun around for a few rotations or when you feel confident that you have set your intention strongly enough for the

---

* Just to clarify: in bed, your sleeping body is paralysed by REM sleep, but in your dream you are spinning around like a spinning top.

technique to work, stop spinning and you should find yourself
in either the same or a newly formed dreamscape with full-level
lucidity.

- It should be noted that spinning can often lead to a false
  awakening, so be sure to apply a reality check immediately after
  this technique.

We've now come to end of our practical techniques section
and we have a toolbox full to the brim of lucid dreaming
techniques and tips. Some people will find one lucidity technique
in particular that really does the job for them, but others may
find themselves trying a different technique each night. Find your
own way around your toolbox and have fun getting to know its
contents.

Before we move into the far-out plains of Part III, we have one
more chapter to explore: embracing the obstacles!

9

Embracing the Obstacles

'If you can find a path with no obstacles,
it probably doesn't lead anywhere.'
FRANK A. CLARK

My first Buddhist teacher, Sogyal Rinpoche, used to say, 'Obstacles are not things that block our path, obstacles are the path.' Never was this truer than on the path of dream work.

There are many obstacles that may seem detrimental to our dream practice – everything from recurring nightmares to missing a night's sleep all together – but I have found that most of these obstacles can be skilfully embraced and some are more like dragons guarding pots of gold and the treasures of lucidity. So, let's meet our dragons…

NIGHTMARES

Many people view nightmares as one of the biggest obstacles to sleep and dream practice, because they create fear and trauma around the process of dreaming, which makes us not want to go to sleep in the first place. But for lucid dreamers, nightmares are opportunities. They can be embraced, transformed and used as mediums of getting lucid. The first time I went on retreat with Rob Nairn, somebody asked him at breakfast how he had slept, to which he replied, 'Very well! I had some wonderful nightmares!' At the time I thought he was mad, but years later I discovered what he meant, because for lucid dreamers nightmares are such good news!

Nightmares usually occur in REM sleep and are typically scenarios in which we are either fighting off or fleeing from terrifying dream characters or situations. Nightmares can occur for a variety of reasons, such as mental and physical illness (and often as a side effect of the drugs used to treat those illnesses), as a result of post-traumatic stress or sometimes just as expressions of a slightly disturbed mind.

Nightmares may be part of what makes us human. Antti Revonsuo, a Finnish scientist who 'collects nightmares', believes that they are rehearsals for the daily struggle to survive. He says, 'Nightmares force us to go through simulated threatening events in order that in the waking world we are more prepared to survive them because we have been training for them in our dreams.'[1] He goes on to say that the reason children frequently have nightmares about wild animals, even if they live in urban areas devoid of such threats, is an inheritance from early humans, who would be faced with life-threatening wild beasts on a daily basis, and that in fact this proves just how vital nightmares were to the evolution of our species. He even speculates, 'Without nightmares there is a good chance that humanity would not exist.'[2]

There is also a good chance that lucid dreaming would not exist either, because scientific research has shown that over a third of all lucid dreams begin as nightmares or anxiety dreams. This is an amazing discovery for lucid dreamers, because it shows that nightmares are a blessing in disguise and that they really are the dragons guarding the gold.

To understand the reason for nightmarish fear preceding lucid dreams so frequently, we first need to understand the reason for fear in the waking state. The biological purpose of fear is to make us scan our surroundings more carefully by boosting selective physical senses and making us more aware of the potential threat or danger. Fear maximizes blood flow to the major muscle groups and to the brain, which increases our sensory perception, allowing us to deal with the potential threat with a heightened level of awareness. Heightened awareness? Maximized blood flow to the brain? Increase of sensory perception? No wonder nightmares lead to lucidity! Everything we need to get lucid is produced as a side effect of fear, so when we experience a fearful nightmare, our awareness is often boosted into lucidity.

Fear within dreams can also help us spot dream signs. In 2009, research at the Erasmus University in Rotterdam found that the experience of fear 'enhances our ability to identify coarse-grain features in preference to fine details'.[3] Of course, if we're being attacked, we don't care if our attacker has wrinkles, we just care about how threatening their movements are! If we apply this to dreaming, we can see that when we experience fear in the dream state our attention will be drawn away from the often deceptively convincing detail of the dreamscape and into a wider visual perspective, which may help us to recognize a previously unnoticed dream sign.

From a Buddhist point of view, nightmares can be a great training ground for fearlessness. Fear is one of the subtlest obstacles on the spiritual path and can often form the basis of major psychological blocks. In the after-death *bardo* state, fear is said to be our biggest obstacle because the *bardo* journey is so intense that for many of us it is an experience of terror, shock and awe. But if we can train in fearlessness through lucid nightmares and create a habit of calm awareness in preference to fear and panic, this will be a huge benefit to us in the after-death *bardo*.

Tibetan medicine actually recommends training in dream yoga so that we can 'recognize the dream as an illusory world in order to pacify negative dreams'[4] and the Tibetan dream yoga teachings recommend that whenever anything of a threatening or nightmarish nature occurs in our dreams, such as being burned by fire, we should become lucid and jump fearlessly into the fire[5] as a way to face our fears, see the emptiness of the dream and prepare for the after-death *bardo*.

Quite simply, nightmares are a blessing for the lucid dreamer and lucid dreaming is a blessing for those who experience nightmares. As we learned earlier, new research on lucid dreaming from the European Science Foundation meeting in 2009 has shown that lucid dreaming is such an effective remedy for working with nightmares that people have the potential to be 'treated by training to dream lucidly'.[6]

NIGHT TERRORS

A night terror is quite different from a nightmare. Whereas nightmares usually occur in REM sleep, night terrors are typically associated with non-dreaming sleep and are 'pure emotional experiences that occur upon awakening from sleep',[7] so they are not actually linked with dreaming at all. They are episodes of extreme panic and fear that occur in the transition from deep sleep to the hypnopompic state, experiences of unadulterated terror, a bit like a night-time panic attack. Subjects may sit bolt upright in bed with their eyes open, screaming, and unable to be roused from this state for several minutes. Those most frequently affected are children aged between three and 12 years old.

Their saving grace is that the subject often has no memory of them and due to the fact that their mind is in the relaxed state of slow-wave sleep, the renowned sleep researcher

William Dement believes they may not be experiencing fear at all, because it is their body that is expressing fright rather than their mind.

> **Charlie says**
>
> *'It's young children who most often experience night terrors, and although this usually freaks their parents out, more than the children themselves, it's not usually a cause for concern. It's thought that night terrors may be caused by the nervous system still maturing and so they often pass as the child grows up.'*

DRUGGED-UP DREAMIN'

There are three main culprits that create the biggest obstacles to sleep and dreaming and most people reading this book will have ingested at least one of them at some point in their life. What are they and how do they affect our sleep and dreams?*

Caffeine

Caffeine, commonly found in soft drinks, diet pills and decongestants, activates parts of the brain that need to be deactivated if we are to sleep. Sleep and wakefulness are influenced by different neurotransmitter signals in the brain, which means that food, drugs and medicines that affect the balance of these signals in turn affect how alert or drowsy we feel and thus how well we sleep. This is old news, but for lucid dreamers the effect of caffeine is not all bad news.

Small amounts of caffeine can make our descent into sleep take longer than usual, meaning that we can stay in the hypnagogic state for longer than usual. This allows us to spend more time

---

* The fourth most widespread legal drug is antidepressant medication, which also often interferes with REM sleep.

getting to know its terrain and its borders. With so many lucid dream induction techniques being dependent on having a good knowledge of the hypnagogic state, if the occasion arises that you have had coffee after dinner and take a while to fall asleep, don't worry – it could be a great opportunity to really engage your hypnagogic state.

There is also the fabled 'caffeine nap', based on research from Loughborough University, which can apparently help people feel more refreshed after an afternoon snooze. The researchers say that because the caffeine in a cup of coffee normally takes about 15 minutes to take effect and 45 minutes to be fully absorbed, it will generally not affect our ability to fall asleep immediately after drinking it[8] but it will often wake us up spontaneously once it starts to kick in, thus negating the grogginess that sometimes follows a nap.

Nicotine

Heavy smokers often sleep very lightly, report reduced amounts of REM sleep and 'may tend to wake up after 3 or 4 hours of sleep due to nicotine withdrawal'.[9] So it seems that smoking cigarettes does little for dream practice. But what about the actual nicotine?

I would like to say that nicotine has no redeeming qualities as far as dream work goes, or as far as anything goes for that matter, but again it's not quite that black and white.

Pure tobacco has been used for generations by shamans to affect the quality of visions and dreams, and wearing nicotine patches while you sleep can have a similar effect. A 2006 study from Monash University, Australia, concluded that: 'More dream reports containing visual imagery occurred while wearing a nicotine patch, and these were rated as more vivid.'[10]

So it seems that going to bed wearing a nicotine patch can induce some dramatic dreaming. But I ask you: is it really worth pumping your sleeping body full of highly addictive nicotine just to have some vivid dreams? Reading a fantasy novel before going to sleep will have much the same effect and probably won't kill you as quickly!

Alcohol

Alcohol is a big obstacle to dream practice because it's a depressant, so it zonks you out,* makes you less likely to be bothered to do any lucid dreaming practice and makes you act unmindfully. And it gives you a hangover.

According to the National Institute of Neurological Disorders and Stroke in the United States, although it may feel as if you are sleeping very deeply if you go to bed drunk, in fact 'alcohol only helps people fall into light sleep, and it also robs people of REM and the deeper, more restorative stages of sleep'.[11]

> **Charlie says**
>
> 'It seems that alcohol is a big no-no for lucidity, right? Perhaps, but I have found that on rare occasions, especially if I am having a drought in my practice, an almost 'homoeopathic amount' of alcohol can actually help. It loosens me up and gives me the confidence to break through my drought. A small glass of wine also allows me to relax and drop my expectations, which can often lead to lucidity.'

Galantamine

And finally, Galantamine. Although this drug is definitely not one of the three most common, within lucid dreaming circles

---

* Cannabis is another drug that really messes with your dream periods and makes dreams harder to recall. I speak from youthful experience. A weed habit is incompatible with a lucid dreaming habit. Sorry, stoners.

it has the number one spot, so it's important that we have a look at it.

Galantamine is a drug sourced from the red spider lily. It is used to treat mild forms of Alzheimer's disease and other memory impairments. It works by increasing the amount of a certain neurotransmitter in the brain that is needed for memory and cognition. It also has an interesting side effect: if you take a dose of Galantamine after about four or five hours of sleep and then go back to sleep with a strong intention to gain lucidity, you are very likely to have a lucid dream.

A couple of years ago I started to come across lucid dreamers who were using Galantamine regularly in order to aid their lucidity. Although I have quite a strong aversion to drug-induced spiritual practice, I thought that I'd better see what all the fuss was about, so I decided to take it three times over a three-month period. I wanted to stay open-minded as to the effects of the drug on lucidity and decided that three trials would allow me to get a pretty good impression of what it was like.

The first night I mistimed the dose and nothing happened, but on the second night, a month later, it did lead to a lucid dream. The lucidity was stable, but it felt really groggy and artificial. On the third and final morning of the trial, something very interesting happened: I took a dose after about four or five hours of sleep, went back to bed and immediately had a false awakening (a dream in which you dream that you have woken up), which I became lucid in. The dreamscape looked exactly like my bedroom, with every detail perfectly replicated apart from one thing: my Buddhist shrine, which sits in a corner of the room, had been vandalized. The symbol of my spirituality had been defaced. I didn't need a dream dictionary to tell me what that meant: my higher self was definitely anti-Galantamine. *(For a full description of this dream, see Dream 11, page 253.)*

If you want to have a lucid dream just for kicks, then Galantamine may seem like a good option, but if you want to have lucid dreams as part of a mind-training programme that aims to foster mindful awareness, wisdom and compassion, then I'm afraid there is no pill that can do that for you. And if there were, would you really want to take it?

To enter into deeper realms of our mind we need that mind to be in its natural, unaltered state, but Galantamine alters that state. It is that simple fact rather than any moral judgement that sets me against taking it.

From a Buddhist point of view, the mind is already pure and we are already a buddha, we just haven't woken up to that fact yet. This means that there is no need to add any drug to our mind in order to reach enlightenment – everything we need is within us already. The ability to lucid dream every night is within us, we just need to keep practising. No drink, drug or psychoactive medicine is needed, just our mind as it is.

Charlie says

'For me, using Galantamine regularly is the equivalent of an athlete taking steroids. It's a shortcut that works well in the short term but will undoubtedly mess with the integrity of your practice in the long run.'

LACK OF SLEEP

The Mindfulness of Dream & Sleep approach embraces all aspects of our journey through sleep, even insomnia. But if you want to learn how to lucid dream specifically, then you do need to be getting some sleep!

Professor Dijk, Professor of Sleep and Physiology at Surrey University, says, 'There is a large body of epidemiological literature suggesting that there are associations between short sleep duration and a number of negative health outcomes including cardiovascular disease… [and] negative effects are noticed in those who regularly sleep for less than six hours, but also those who regularly sleep more than 10 hours',[12] which seems to confirm the standard advice to sleep for about seven or eight hours per night.*

> **Charlie says**
>
> 'Sleep is a bit like calories. If you are doing a lot of hard physical work then you may need more calories. Just as there is a recommended daily calorie intake for men and women based on the average person living the average lifestyle, so there is with hours of sleep. But I am yet to meet an average person, so don't let anyone tell you how much or how little sleep you need. Only you know that.'

'So, what about Margaret Thatcher?' you may ask. 'She used to get by perfectly well on a tiny amount of sleep!' This is true. There are some people who seem to be able to go to bed late and rise early, surviving on as little as three hours of sleep most nights. There are two types of such people. One is comprised of long-term spiritual practitioners who are engaging in so many hours of deep-level meditation during the day that their need for sleep is partially negated.** Needless to say, Margaret Thatcher was not one of these. She was the second type, the so-called 'sleepless élite'…

In 2009 the University of California discovered a gene variant affecting about 1% of the population, which allowed them to

---

* I would change this advice to seven or eight hours per 24-hour cycle, because the eight hours don't have to be all in one go.

** This is due to a phenomenon called 'eyes-open delta wave' in which meditators reach the delta-wave brain state while awake in meditation. This allows them to engage the restorative qualities of deep sleep without sleeping.

survive on just a few hours' sleep per night with little or no detriment to their health.[13] This 'sleepless élite' had certain common traits, such as a faster than average metabolism, unusual circadian rhythms and an unusually high pain threshold. Although many sleep-deprived, overworked optimists like to think that they are members of this élite group, most are not. There is one way to know for certain: you don't feel constantly tired and you never feel the need for a weekend lie-in.

REM Rebound

So, how can we actually embrace the obstacle of lack of sleep? The answer lies in 'REM rebound'. This phenomenon is based on the fact that if a person misses a whole night's worth of REM sleep, their next sleep cycle will contain much more REM in order to 'pay back the debt' from the previous night.

Dream periods usually last between five minutes and 60 minutes in length, but once you throw some REM rebound into the mix, you might find that you can extend those REM periods considerably. REM rebound can be great for lucid dreaming, because more REM sleep means more chances of lucidity.

Charlie says

'*REM rebound is a phenomenon that I made use of many times when I was on tour with the hip-hop group I was in. We would often be performing in clubs late at night and then be travelling the next day, so sometimes I would go for 48 hours with very little sleep. I'm not saying that everybody should go out partying till 6 a.m. just to have a lucid dream, but if you do happen to miss a night's sleep then be ready for action the next night, because the REM periods will be coming thick and fast!*'

Although the next three obstacles cannot be directly embraced on our path of mindful dreams and sleep, it is worth being aware of how they work. They are the three sleep phenomena that I get asked about most regularly when I'm teaching.

SLEEPWALKING

Sleepwalking is not, as often believed, the acting out of the physical movements corresponding to dream content, because it takes place in the earlier stages of the sleep cycle, often during non-REM sleep before REM dreaming has occurred, so sleepwalkers aren't dreaming. Sleepwalking is a parasomnia most commonly experienced by children or by people with high levels of stress, anxiety or illness, and can be genetically influenced as well.

Although the motor systems are inhibited during all the stages of sleep (and of course totally inhibited during REM sleep), sometimes the movement systems in the sub-cortical brain tissue become activated during non-REM sleep (which is when this motor system inhibition is less active), leading to unconscious automatic movement.[14] The complexity of this automatic movement differs from person to person and so we could postulate that people who, for example, do a lot of cycling may find that the act of cycling is an automatic enough process to allow them to sleep cycle through their sleep cycle.

Charlie says

'A woman in Sydney, Australia, had apparently been regularly sleepwalking out of her house at night. This went on for months until one night her husband saw it happening, followed her and caught her having sex with a stranger! Although I have full sympathy for the couple involved, I can't help wondering whether she'd come up with that alibi before or after her husband had caught her having sex with another man?'

SLEEPTALKING

A soliloquy is a direct address from a character in a play to the audience, revealing their true feelings, so it is no surprise that somniloquy is the name given to sleeptalking. Sleeptalking, like sleepwalking, is a parasomnia, but a much more common one, with up to 50 per cent of children reported to talk in their sleep. This drops to 5 per cent of adults.[15]

Sleeptalking is mainly associated with non-dreaming sleep, but can also occur during REM sleep due to something called 'motor breakthrough', which is when the sleep-paralysis function of REM sleep is momentarily 'broken through', leading to words that are being spoken in the dream being spoken out loud.*

REM SLEEP BEHAVIOUR DISORDER

What used to be mistaken for a type of sleepwalking is now recognized as a distinct condition with neurological roots of a much more ominous nature. This is the condition known as REM sleep behaviour disorder (RBD), which occurs when subjects physically act out their dreams as they are dreaming them.

When someone is woken from an episode of RBD, their dream description will usually fit with the physical movements that they were making, whether it's fighting off an attacker or smoking a cigarette. But how does it work?

During REM sleep, an area of the brain called the pons causes the body to be in a state of physical paralysis so that we don't act out our dreams. However, if the pons is damaged, it may cease to do this and so we will act out our dreams.

In July 2008 a 59-year-old Welshman with a history of sleepwalking and RBD-like behaviour stopped taking his

---

* The respiratory system is not paralysed during REM sleep, and because speaking is in part caused by air from the respiratory system flowing over the vocal cords, it's not surprising that sleeptalking can happen quite easily.

medication and tragically killed his wife while he was dreaming of fighting off attackers.[16] This isn't the only possible problem. RBD in middle-aged men can often be a precursor to Parkinson's disease, and other subjects may have had their serotonin and dopamine levels upset by the use of antidepressant drugs such as serotonin uptake inhibitors, which in turn affect the inhibition of motor systems during sleep.

Some people do occasionally thrash around in their sleep. If it only happens now and then, not to worry, but if you or a loved one regularly move around while asleep and if your movements match your dream recall, it might be worth getting this checked out with a doctor, because it could be a sign of something that requires attention.

'I JUST CAN'T DO IT!'

The final obstacle to lucid dreaming that we are going to look at is pure fantasy, I assure you. The inability to have lucid dreams is as much of an illusion as the dreams themselves. If you dream, you can lucid dream – it's as simple as that.

I've taught people who have had their first ever lucid dream after a 30-minute drop-in workshop at a music festival, but I've also taught people who've done eight-week courses and weekend retreats, read all the books on the subject and still struggled to get lucid regularly. Lucid dreaming may not be particularly easy to learn, but in all the years that I've taught it, I've yet to encounter a person who *cannot* learn how to do it.

We're all working from wonderfully different starting-points of mental capacity, dream recall and motivation, and this leads to a plethora of different successes and challenges along the path of lucid dreaming. Nevertheless, I can say with certainty that if you apply sustained effort with strong motivation, your first lucid dream will definitely come, and once you have tasted lucidity for the first time, it will be much easier to taste it again.

'The chains of habit are often too weak to be felt until they are too strong to be broken',[17] so don't feel discouraged if it seems that you are making slow progress, because you may be just one more night away from your tipping point, a breakthrough moment that will make all the hard work seem worth its weight in gold. Lucidity training is cumulative and each night of training (regardless of whether you become lucid or not) fills up your lucidity tank drop by drop. You might be just one drop away from a lucid dream.

My teacher Rob Nairn once said, 'Although Charlie talks about lucidity like it's an everyday occurrence, just to have one intentional lucid dream in your lifetime is an achievement.' This is very true, but what he didn't mention was that lucidity isn't always an everyday occurrence for me anyway. If I'm in training and feeling confident, I can have up to five fully lucid dreams each night, but every now and again I will go weeks without any lucidity and feel like a total fraud! I lose my confidence and start to doubt myself. Because I doubt myself, I stop training. Because I stop training, my lucidity tank runs dry. And finally I feel that I've lost my ability forever, I'll be forced to quit teaching and catastrophe is looming!

How do I get myself back on track when I fall into this kind of melodramatic ego trap? I relax, I stop trying and I make friends with my feelings of failure. I rekindle my inspiration by reading a new book on the subject or watching a dream-themed film, and most importantly I talk to someone. I open up about my fears and doubts and feelings of failure, knowing that this will free them up and allow my lucid awareness to flow back to me naturally. It always does.

Besides, it's not just about getting lucid, anyway. Lucid dreaming is only one part of the Mindfulness of Dream & Sleep approach. After a couple of years of teaching pure lucid dreaming I saw that it was an inherently limited method in that it could only be practised in the two or three hours we spent dreaming each night. That's why Rob Nairn and I came up with the idea of Mindfulness of Dream & Sleep, because we saw that lucid dreaming needed to be taught as part of a holistic approach to dream work that used all aspects of sleep for psychological growth, not just dreaming.

One of the major problems with lucid dream practice is the name 'lucid dreaming'. The aim is in the name, which leads people to think that they are outright failures if they don't achieve this aim. Let me clarify… In the game of baseball, the aim is to score home runs, but the name of the game isn't 'home run ball', it's baseball. Why? Because baseball is about proceeding through the bases, not just about hitting the home runs. It's the same with lucid dreaming. Just as you can be a great baseball player without having hit many home runs, so you can be a great Mindfulness of Dream & Sleep practitioner without having had many lucid dreams. You might be a great hypnopompic mindfulness meditator, or have great dream recall, or be able to maintain awareness into NREM sleep. All these are great attributes to have on the playing field of lucidity and yet none of them are determined by having a lucid dream.

A lady on my first course told me, 'I haven't even had my first lucid dream yet, but I can say for sure that the act of sleeping will never be the same again. I can't unknow what I've learned: about the sleep stages, the process of dreaming, the hypnagogic states… Falling asleep will never be the same again.'

The experience of that student was actually more important to me than the experiences of all the students who were lucid from week one, because what it showed me was that the process of learning how to bring awareness into dream and sleep had profoundly changed a lifetime of habitual tendency –

something which is of far more benefit than just having a one-off lucid dream.

The most important thing to remember is this: don't *just* fall asleep. Try to do something, however small, each and every night. If you're struggling with lucidity, train in your daytime reality checks. If you're struggling with dream recall, work on your daily mindfulness. If you're too tired at night to stay aware, take a nap during the day. There are so many ways in which you can engage this practice, so don't put it off, do something today. Make a change, however small. For, in the words of the poet John Greenleaf Whittier, 'For all the sad words of tongue or pen, the saddest are these: it might have been.'[18]

Make your next sleep the first sleep of the rest of your life.

PART III
GERMINATION

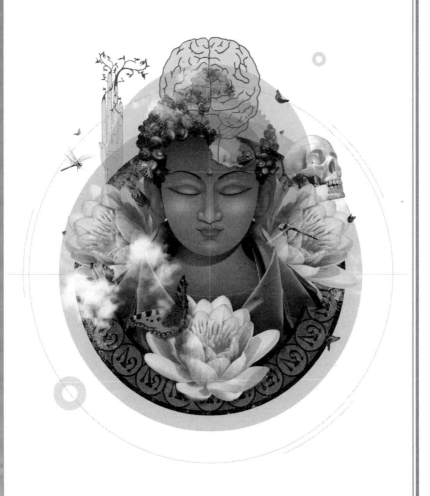

PART III

GERMINATION

10

Blurring the Boundaries

'Deep into that darkness peering, long I stood there,
wondering, fearing, doubting, dreaming dreams
no mortal ever dared to dream before.'
EDGAR ALLAN POE

The lucid dream is a unique state of consciousness in which we gain access to a depth of mind unfathomable to most people who haven't yet experienced it. And once lucid, we can use our increased energetic capacity as a springboard to dive through the boundaries of the dream into something quite different.

Moving through these boundaries is the germination of the practice. We descend into the depths of our own mind, and if we keep on swimming, deeper and deeper down, we may find that the boundary between our personal consciousness and universal consciousness begins to blur. Freud famously popularized the iceberg theory of consciousness in which a small percentage of our mind is above the surface, conscious and tangible, and the majority below the surface, unconscious and rarely accessible. Through lucid dreaming we not only gain access to the vast expanse of the iceberg below the surface but also to the infinite sea of awareness in which the iceberg floats.

A lucid dream is a partially permeable membrane through which we can access states beyond our personal mindstream. Through a form of conscious osmosis we can leave the limitations of our own mind behind and flow into the limitless awareness of the void.

PROPHETIC DREAMS

A dreamer is one who can only find his way by moonlight, and his punishment is that he sees the dawn before the rest of the world.
Oscar Wilde

Within Tibetan Buddhism, prophetic dreams are classed as a type of clarity dream and have been systematically used by realized masters to help find reincarnations and to inform themselves of future events. Nevertheless, for the most part it's believed that 'although certain prophecies of future happenings may be true, mostly they will not be'[1] and that to believe that all of your dreams are prophetic is often a sign of an overactive ego. So it is advised within the teachings to check your motivation carefully before you claim to have had a prophetic dream.

In Western culture, our view on prophetic dreams is slightly more inconclusive, but it's a subject that has been close to our heart since our culture began. In fact the propagation of the Christian culture into the West can be attributed in part to a prophetic dream. The Roman Emperor Constantine dreamed he was visited by Jesus Christ on the night before a big battle and then attributed his victory to the dream.[2] Apparently this led him to make Christianity the new religion of the Roman Empire.

More recently, both Freud and Jung acknowledged dream telepathy.[3] In *Man and his Symbols,* Jung comments that the unconscious has a facility to predict future events not due to any mystical aptitude but rather to the vast amount of information it stores:'Dreams sometimes announce certain situations long before they actually happen. This is not necessarily a form of precognition... What we fail to see consciously is frequently perceived by our unconscious, which can pass the information on through dreams.'[4] It is as if the data that the unconscious stores (but the conscious mind ignores) can be used to create predictive algorithms of possible future outcomes. Sometimes these predictions come true. This is not precognition, it's more like preparation.

Over a third of British people claim to have had at least one dream in which they prophesied a future event[5], and although there is a lot of research that disproves most seemingly prophetic dreams as contrived coincidences noticed after the actual event, there is just too much data in favour of prophetic dreams to ignore them completely. In 1997 a paper published in the *Journal of the American Society for Psychical Research* proved that 37 of a supposed 51 precognitive dreams gathered for the study could be objectively substantiated.[6] Throughout my own research into this topic I've been shocked by just how much scientific data there is supporting the possibility of prophetic dreams.

Among the most memorable were two cases presented at the Scientific and Medical Network conference at Winchester University in 2011. One was that of an American woman who kept dreaming that she had breast cancer even though the scans found nothing. She eventually paid for invasive surgery and a tiny cyst was found, too small to show up on the scan, which had all the hallmarks of turning malignant in the future.[7] Then there was the case of a group of stock market investors led by a dream psychologist called Arthur Bernard, who ended up making a sales profit of US$1.6 million in 1998 after one of them had a prophetic dream about buying shares in an obscure biotech firm.[8] In the words of one of the presenters at the conference,

Dr Larry Dossey, 'We are way beyond anecdotes here, the evidence is just too strong to ignore.'[9]

> **Charlie says**
>
> *'I know what you're probably thinking: If people can have dreams of the future, why don't they dream of the winning lottery numbers? Well, actually they do! In one well-documented example, a woman in America won the lottery twice after dreaming of the winning numbers!*[10]

Prophetic dreams can be split into two main categories: precognitive dreams (pre = before, cognitive = knowing); and premonition dreams (pre = before, monition = warning). But how do they actually work? Dr Larry Dossey, a well-known pioneer of science-based research into spirituality, considers that we may well be genetically endowed for premonition dreams, as they would seem to aid our survival.[11] He believes that prophetic dreams may be a type of innate but often dormant preventative medicine that resides within all of us, and he even cites examples in which his stint as a Vietnam War surgeon led to a series of premonition dreams, some of which even saved his life.

The Nobel physicist Brian Josephson says, 'It's not clear in physics why we *can't* see the future,'[12] and although frustratingly inconclusive, the closest to a scientific explanation we have for prophetic dreams is that they may be caused by our consciousness engaging in non-local communication through the vast quantum interconnectivity of reality in which time, and thus past and future events, are relative. Nobody knows for sure, but then nobody knows for sure what dark energy is either, and that makes up 70 per cent of the known universe.[13] Perhaps for now we will have to accept that although we don't have a cast-iron explanation for how this phenomenon works, we do have some pretty convincing examples that it does work.

How Can We Encourage Prophetic Dreams?

It has been said that 'premonitions are our birth right. Our capacity for them is part of our original equipment, something that comes factory installed.'[14] So, if precognitive dreams are natural, why don't most of us have them regularly?

The reason may be because most of us aren't in tune with our own nature or our own dreams, so we aren't tuned into the wavelength on which they are broadcast. Some people believe that our natural capacity for precognitive dreaming has deteriorated due to our use of modern communications technology, which has led to our telepathic muscles atrophying from lack of use, but I believe the truth is more straightforward: our sixth sense has withered not only from lack of use but also from lack of attention. Most people are simply not interested in it.

Once we inhabit the awareness of our subtle energies and sixth-sense capacity through mind-training practices, however, or even simply open ourselves up to the possibility that they exist, we become less disconnected from them and less limited. So, we can help remedy our precognitive dreaming limitations by practising energy work such as chakra-based meditation, *tai chi* or *chi gong*, as well as keeping a dream diary in order to pay attention to our dreaming mind. These practices will help boost the power of our extra-sensory awareness and help deepen the connection to our subtle energies and to our dreaming mind.

The unconscious is far more likely to offer a precognitive dream to someone who is already in tune with their dream life than to someone with no dream recall or interest in their dreams. However, the most direct way to open up our potential for precognitive dreaming is to become lucid. Due to the refined level of consciousness we enter into through the lucid dream state, we become more attuned to the innate capacity of our sixth sense, which is often pushed aside in the waking state by the other, more dominant, five senses. As we learned earlier, the lucid dream state is a 'thin' place, meaning that its boundaries are semi-permeable. While lucid, the dream yoga teachings say that we also have seven times the potential mental clarity that we have in the waking state.[15] This means that we can ask for information which can be invited back through the semi-permeable membrane of the dream state and deciphered with seven times our waking clarity. By intentionally calling out for future information within a lucid dream, I have seen detailed images of people I have yet to meet, been warned of two deaths (which tragically did take place, regardless of my premonition) and even received winning numbers on the lottery.*

If future information can be invited into the lucid dreaming mind, perhaps it can be sent out from it, too? In 2011 I conducted an informal experiment into dream telepathy with the members of the monthly Lucid Dreaming Forum in London. I was to get lucid sometime within the next 30 nights, visualize the forum members and tell them where on my body I had a birthmark.

Funnily enough, I ended up forgetting about the experiment and it was only on the night before the next month's forum that I remembered it. That night I became lucid, visualized as many of the forum members as I could recollect and then called out, 'Right hip! The birthmark is on my right hip!' I even visualized the birthmark and projected it up into the sky in the lucid dream as I repeated, 'The birthmark is on my right hip!'

The next day I asked the dream forum members if anyone had received a dream or any other indication as to where my birthmark was. After a good minute of silence and polite smiles, I continued, 'OK. Well, not to worry, but the birthmark is actually on…' and then suddenly one of the members, who had been looking through his dream diary, called out, 'Right hip! It's on your

---

* I gave the money I won to charity. In fact that was part of the deal, because when I went into the lucid dream I called out, 'Give me the winning lottery numbers! If I win, I'll give the money to charity!'

right hip, isn't it? I think it might be on your right ankle, but the dream says it's definitely on your right hip."*

But all this precognitive dreaming stuff is for nothing unless we have some way of telling if this dream information is the real deal, right? How do we know?

It is said that although the vast majority of dreams aren't premonition dreams, if you do have one it will leave such a lasting mental and possibly even physical remnant afterwards that you'll be in no doubt.[16] Remember, precognitive dreams may be a kind of evolutionary trait, so your gut instinct will be really trying to make sure that you get the warning message. Also, the dream will seem very different from dreams you've had before and it may recur until you have taken on board its message.[17] If you have a premonition dream, you'll know about it.

SLEEP PARALYSIS

From the Japanese *kanashibari* (fastened in metal), to the African 'witch riding your back' to *incubus/succubus* myths of the West, the phenomenon of the brain waking up from sleep but the body staying paralysed has been mythologized within almost every culture. Thankfully, we now know that sleep paralysis is a neurologically explained phenomenon, which helps to put the demonic myths of the past to bed.

Sleep paralysis is caused by one of the three REM sleep systems (muscular paralysis), staying engaged when the other two (sensory blockade and cortical activation) have been disengaged, meaning that while your brain has partially woken up and your senses are taking in partial sensory input, your physical body cannot move.

Sleep paralysis most commonly occurs during the hypnopompic state, but sometimes in the hypnagogic, too,

---

* Weirdly, I do actually have a birthmark on my right ankle, too.

and is an often hallucinatory experience in which the dreamer may feel totally awake and the room that they wake up in may look exactly the same as it normally does, but due to the brain's momentary engagement in both the dream state and waking state there may be hallucinatory images superimposed over the normal field of vision and there are often loud audio hallucinations, too.

This can be a terrifying experience, but it is a terror that is mostly rooted in the mystery of the situation. Waking up and feeling that your body is paralysed leads to intense fear, which can also lead to hyperventilation, which in turn can lead to a feeling of weight on your chest. This often goes together with hypnagogic hallucinations, which are aural and visual dream aspects superimposed on the waking world. Now add to the mix the fact that sleep paralysis is often accompanied by a form of hyperacusis (a condition in which sounds become amplified and distorted) and the genital arousal that often accompanies the REM sleep we have just come from, and we can see why in earlier times possession by a sexualized demon often seemed to be the best explanation.*

Charlie says

'I woke up in my bed and looked around the room. I was unable to move and there was a dark ominous presence around me. There was a pressure on my chest. I felt a scaly hand cover my face. It had claws. I could feel them across my cheekbones. I began to panic. Someone was in my room. Alien life forms were about to abduct me! Then suddenly it hit me: Hang on, this is sleep paralysis! It's all a hallucination! This is so cool!'

---

* Some researchers believe that alien abductions can often be put down to misinterpreted sleep paralysis. If you look at the timings and the actual subjective reports, the argument does seem to hold some weight.

If you want to break free from sleep paralysis while you're experiencing it then the best course of action is to relax and exhale one long breath through your front teeth, making a sound similar to letting air out of a tyre. This relaxation of the respiratory system will help to disengage the paralysis mechanism and bring you back into your rational mind. Think of yourself as a diver who knows that they must come up to the surface slowly and without panic if they are to avoid the bends. Just relax, breathe out and follow the bubbles to the surface.

Although sleep paralysis may seem to go on for hours, it rarely lasts for more than a couple of minutes and is quite a common occurrence. It isn't anything to be feared or dreaded. Most probably you haven't been possessed by demons, you aren't going mad and there aren't any dark forces in your bedroom. You are safe, and all that is happening is that your brain has woken up before your body has.

Those training in Mindfulness of Dream & Sleep should be grateful for sleep paralysis, because during it you have one foot in the dream world and one in the waking world – the perfect state from which to drop back into a dream lucidly and a very interesting state to observe mindfully.*

---

* Sleep paralysis can become quite common among people who are learning to dream lucidly (due to the increased awareness of the hypnopompic they develop) and is often actually a sign of progression along the path.

FALSE AWAKENINGS

All that we see, or seem to see, is but a dream within a dream.
EDGAR ALLAN POE

Charlie says

'I woke up in my bed and reached for the bedside lamp. I flicked the switch, but it wouldn't turn on. The bulb had blown. I sat up, unplugged the lamp and unscrewed the bulb. I shook it and heard the rattle of the blown filament. I looked closely and could see the fragments of the blown filament inside the glass bulb. I reached over to replace the bulb and suddenly I realized that I don't even have a bedside lamp. No way! I thought. Then I woke up in my bed – for real this time.'

Welcome to the weird world of false awakenings…

A false awakening is the experience of dreaming that we've woken up when we are in fact still dreaming. We might dream that we've woken up in our bed as normal, with our bedroom looking identical to real life, until suddenly we wake up from this dream within a dream to actual waking reality. Some people even have multiple false awakenings in which they dream of waking up, getting out of bed and then waking up again. So they get out of bed again, reflect on their previous false awakening and then suddenly they wake up again, for real this time: a dream within a dream within a dream.

Although they sometimes happen spontaneously, false awakenings often manifest when people start doing lucid dream training and frequently occur after a fully lucid dream. They are very strange experiences and have been described by some researchers as 'a lucid dream – minus the lucidity'.[18]

The 'reality' of a false awakening often seems absolutely identical to waking reality, including a perfectly detailed carbon copy of our bedroom without any aspect seeming dreamlike at all, but if we get into the habit of doing a reality check as soon as we wake up, we can transform every false awakening we have into a lucid dream.

Becoming lucid within a false awakening can be one of the most bizarre experiences in the lucid dream canon, because the reality that we find ourselves in is so utterly undreamlike – a mentally constructed doppelgänger of reality – that it calls into question the very nature of the waking state.

In late 2010, as part of my research for this section of the book I set out intentionally to have as many false awakenings as I could. I managed to have seven fully lucid false awakenings in a row or a 'dream within a dream within a dream within a dream...' – you get the idea. Each successive false awakening seemed to bring me closer to waking reality. The first false awakening was quite dreamy, and I could fly about and affect the dream easily through mental intent, but each subsequent awakening brought with it a decrease in volitional influence and an increase in the 'normality' of the dreamscape. By the sixth false awakening, hand reality checks were barely working, I was unable to fly and my ability to transform the dreamscape was very weak. With each successive false awakening I seemed to be coming closer and closer to waking reality. This made me wonder if our waking reality is the final level of wakefulness or just another false awakening in which we are yet to get lucid? With spiritual realization being so often referred to as 'awakening from a dream', perhaps this isn't such a crazy proposition.

False awakenings are undoubtedly weird boundary experiences, but not nearly as weird as our next subject...

OUT-OF-BODY EXPERIENCES (OBEs)

'Toto, I have a feeling we're not in Kansas anymore.'
DOROTHY, *THE WIZARD OF OZ*

An out-of-body experience typically involves the subjective separation or dislocation of personal consciousness from the physical body. This often allows the consciousness or sense of self to explore not only physical waking reality but seemingly alternate dimensions of reality as well. Although there are dozens of variations, the classic OBE involves our sense of self shifting out of our physical body and looking back to see it lying below. This type of dislocation of consciousness has been well documented as a neurological response to shock, intense stress, trauma or anaesthetic, and yet full OBEs have yet to be accepted by mainstream science.

Scientific studies in 2010 have shown that the idea that our sense of self is fixed in our body is a misconception anyway. If the body's sense of spatial awareness is sufficiently confused by receiving contradictory input then the sense of self will locate itself in a close but separate location to the body.

The study that best proved this point was run by researchers at the Karolinska Institute in Stockholm.[19] They conducted an experiment aimed at creating the illusion, and physical sensation, of having a third arm. In five separate laboratory experiments, 154 volunteers were seated with their hands on a table and a rubber arm was placed next to their right arm. A sheet covered their shoulders and elbows, creating the illusion that they had three arms. The scientists then gently brushed the real and fake hands at the end of those arms. Sometimes the brushing occurred simultaneously, sometimes separately. When it occurred at the same time, the subjects would report feeling the sensation in the rubber hand as well and even feeling as if they had two right hands. Their sense of personal self had partially left or at least expanded from the constraints of their physical body to include an inanimate object, the fake rubber arm.

You might be thinking, *If we can relocate the conscious awareness of a limb to outside ourselves, could we do so with our entire body?* It seems that we can, as researchers in France have used the rubber arm experiment to inspire a kind of rubber body experiment which has demonstrated that 'there is a systematic relationship between the body-part illusion and full-body illusion'[20] which allows the sense of self to relocate into another *full-body* form.

Although these experiments are more indicative of bodily illusions than OBEs, they are still an interesting way to show that although our consciousness is *habitually* limited to our physical body, it is not *exclusively* limited. But what I'd like to focus on now is the kind of intentional OBE or 'astral projection' which most often occurs in or around the boundaries of falling asleep and dreaming: a sleep-initiated OBE.* In these experiences beginners sometimes feel intense rushing vibrations as they pass through the hypnagogic or hypnopompic states and experience their consciousness being separated, often forcibly, from their physical body. Once their consciousness has been separated, they might find themselves in an energy duplicate of their body or sometimes as a point of awareness seemingly floating around anywhere from their local environment to an apparently alternate reality. But are they really dislocated from their physical body or are they just imagining it all? To explore this question, let us first (through gritted teeth) offer the stage to the sceptics and look at the argument against sleep-initiated OBEs.

Many people claim to have had OBEs pretty much exclusively around the time of falling asleep and waking up, or often in the early hours of the morning – prime times for lucid dreams, sleep

---

* 'Sleep-initiated OBE' is a bit of a misnomer because in some cases the subjects are more in a state of heightened awareness than a sleep state, but it seems the best label to use here nonetheless.

paralysis and false awakenings. This has led some sceptics to classify sleep-initiated OBEs as nothing more than unrecognized aspects of these three dream phenomena. Let's look at each of them in a little more detail.

Lucid Dreams without the Lucidity?

There are three key factors that seem to suggest that some sleep-initiated OBEs are just a type of unrecognized lucid dream: timing, location and experience.

The timing of these OBEs — mostly around falling asleep at night or in a nap — can of course seem a bit suspect. The location can, too. With over 80 per cent of all reported OBEs occurring when the subject was lying down,[21] often in bed, some people deduce that it is 80 per cent possible that most OBEs are just a type of dream.

Furthermore, many OBEs are described as an experience of being fully conscious within a totally realistic three-dimensional reality that is 'just too realistic to have been a dream'. This is a common reaction to our first few lucid dreams.

So it seems that there is quite an argument for the possibility that the only difference between a night-time 'OBEer' and a lucid dreamer is that the lucid dreamer knows that they're inside their own head whereas the OBEer believes that they are experiencing a reality outside themselves. Some researchers believe that most sleep-initiated OBEers are simply lucid dreamers who haven't become fully lucid yet.

In a lucid dream we may find ourselves in a seemingly autonomous fully functional other world which is very different from waking reality. We might be able to fly, and communicate with strange autonomous beings, and receive teachings from sources of expanded consciousness and/or our own higher self, but all the time we are fully aware that we are inside our own imagination and having a lucid dream. However convincing this 'other world' seems, a lucid dreamer knows that it is all just a construct of their dreaming mind.

But imagine if we were to engage these kinds of actions within the pre-lucid state, a state in which we are yet to fully accept that we are in fact dreaming. Without the 'Aha!' moment of full lucidity, we would be interacting with the content of our mind just as in a lucid dream, but we would believe it to be occurring outside our mind and thus outside our body.

Dream researcher Paul Devereux believes that it is very simple: lucid dreamers know that they are experiencing a dream within their mind, while those who label the experience an OBE take the dream to be waking reality.

Just Sleep Paralysis or False Awakenings?

Another argument against sleep-initiated OBEs is that they are actually a type of misinterpreted sleep paralysis. Stephen LaBerge says that 'to the sleep researcher, these strange phenomena are remarkably reminiscent of sleep paralysis'[22] and that because OBEs so often occur at precisely the same times that we would expect sleep paralysis to occur, this is an option that we definitely need to consider.

He goes on to say that some of the experiences that subjects report during sleep paralysis, such as a feeling of being separated from their body, a hissing in the ears and a roaring sensation in the head, 'appear to be much like the OBE sensations of vibrations, strange noises, and drifting away from the physical body'.[23] In addition to this, experiences of dark entities and otherworldly beings are sometimes as common to reports of sleep paralysis as they are to OBEs, so without validated evidence to the contrary it seems as though this argument might be difficult to disprove altogether.

The final argument that the sceptics throw down is that in sleep-initiated OBEs in which the subject seems to be experiencing actual waking reality (sometimes called a 'Locale I' OBE), are they really just experiencing a false awakening? In a false awakening we often find ourselves in a mentally constructed carbon copy of our sleeping area that seems to all intents and purposes to be waking reality. But if we become lucid within a false awakening, we recognize that although it may look exactly like waking reality we are in fact still inside our own head.

Without reality checks to tell whether we were dreaming or not it would be very difficult to accept that we weren't in waking reality when we were in a false awakening, so maybe the only difference between this and the illusion of a Locale I OBE is the realization of lucidity?

The reason that I have given the arguments of the sceptics so much space here is that I used to be an OBE sceptic, too – until I had my first proper OBE that is. I was sure that most OBEs were just pre-lucid dreams, and in fact I still believe now that many people are mixing up the two, but once I had experienced proper OBEs (both through transition into sleep and while wide awake), I realized that the only reason some people might be confused between a lucid dream and an OBE was that they hadn't had sufficient experience of either one.

So let's take a closer look at OBEs and see how they form one of the best-documented aspects of consciousness exploration yet to be accepted by mainstream science.

Proof of OBEs

Much of the proof of OBEs being the real deal (and not just some sort of dream phenomenon) comes not from the mystics who are claiming to have them but from the scientists who are trying to disprove them. Scientifically speaking, lucid dreams and OBEs are both psychologically and physiologically distinct. In the early 80s, the Australian professor Harvey Irwin conducted a thorough comparative study[24] of lucid dreams and sleep-initiated OBEs, which concluded that most OBEs were unlike lucid dreams because during an OBE the brainwave patterns would often show alpha activity but hardly ever any REM, meaning that whatever the subjects were actually doing, they were definitely not dreaming.

To add to this neuroscientific evidence, we can offer the sceptics some more from scientifically oriented psychology. Keith Harary, Executive Director of the Institute for Advanced Psychology in Portland, Oregon, has done some excellent all-round OBE studies. Although he still believes that nobody actually knows quite what an OBE is, he proved under scientific conditions that his pet cat displayed significantly more settled behaviour when he had guided his sense of self to its location during several randomly timed OBEs than when his sense of self (or whatever he believed was being projected out of his body) was not with the cat.

But what about the physicists? Surely they can't believe in all this stuff? On the contrary, some of the most convincing experiments into OBEs were conducted by a nuclear physicist called Dr Thomas Campbell. In his book *My Big TOE*, Campbell describes the process through which he validated his OBEs:

> *'Somebody would write down a random number and we would read it while our bodies lay asleep. Then they would erase it and write another one, and so on and on. We went places – to people's homes – and saw what they were doing, then called them or talked to them the next day to check it out for validation.'[25]*

Campbell collected some of the most convincing data for the OBE as a real phenomenon distinct from dreams, and his position as a respected nuclear physicist gave his data even more kudos.

And then of course there is the work of Robert Monroe. If you still have any doubts about the validity of OBEs after reading this chapter then read his seminal work, *Journeys Out of the Body*. In this he describes dozens of personal OBE accounts meticulously analysed for inconsistencies and far too detailed to be the work of a fraud.

Monroe went on to set up the non-profit Monroe Institute, which gathered such hard proof of the validity of OBEs that the former director of the Intelligence and Security Command of the US Army sent his personnel there for training. I know that seems hard to believe, but it is true. In fact, US Army documents declassified in 1995 reveal that the US government invested millions of dollars over 20 years in several top-secret projects which aimed to use OBE and remote viewing as a way to spy on the Russian military during the Cold War. One of these 'psychic spies' (a man named Joe McMoneagle) was even awarded the Legion of Merit by the US Military for his discovery of a Russian submarine in 1979 through remote viewing.

Although there is no conclusive agreement on how they happen, OBEs arising from stress, trauma or anaesthesia have been verified, so why is it so hard for us to believe that they could be induced at will or via the gateway of sleep? For years scientists believed that lucid dreaming was 'a paradoxical impossibility' and that it was in fact just a misdiagnosed form of micro-awakening. Perhaps the argument that a sleep-initiated OBE is simply a misinterpreted dream phenomenon is just as weak?

We cannot dismiss the hundreds of verified accounts from people who have been able to project their consciousness out of their physical body just because we haven't agreed on the scientific explanation for how they do it. That's exactly what we did with remote viewers, meditators and self-hypnotists before Western science eventually caught up with them.

The scientific evidence for OBEs is just too overwhelming to ignore, but even without it there are many discernible differences between OBEs and lucid dreams which we can use ourselves to differentiate the two.

> **Charlie says**
>
> *'Lucid dreams require that the subject is in REM dreaming sleep, but OBEs can of course be engaged from the waking state. In fact you don't even need to be lying down to have an OBE, let alone be asleep. My friend the OBE expert Graham Nicholls told me of an OBE he had once which began while he was walking to his kitchen. He felt the energy shift begin as he entered his kitchen and as it increased he went to lie down on the floor to allow the full experience to manifest.'*

HOW TO SPOT AN OBE

I've had hundreds of lucid dreams over the past 13 years and so I know the lucid dream state well enough to know when I'm in it and when I'm not. When I have an OBE I'm definitely not in the lucid dream state as I know it. They feel as different as water and ice – the same essence perhaps but totally different forms.

There are loads of ways to tell the difference between a sleep-initiated OBE and a lucid dream, but here are a few of my top tells.

Entry

The entry into an OBE is often very different from that of a lucid dream. There are two main ways to enter a lucid dream: either you enter consciously, in which case you watch the hypnagogic imagery layer until gradually the dreamscape is fully formed and you are lucid within it, or alternatively you may be in the dream for some time before having the 'Aha!' moment and becoming lucid. Entry into an OBE is very different. If you enter the OBE state through the transition into sleep (much like the FAC technique), rather than the gradual layering of the hypnagogic imagery, you may experience intense vibrations, loud audio hallucinations and a rushing sensation as your consciousness is forcibly shifted out of your body. When you first experience this, you'll be in no doubt that you're not entering a lucid dream.

Another way to enter the OBE state is from within a lucid dream. Once you are lucid, there are certain techniques you can apply *within* the dream which will result in being transported from it (often sucked upwards or pulled forward forcefully) and into the OBE state.

How can you tell that you're not merely in another lucid dream? Because reality checks and other lucid dream indicators won't function in the same way.*

Embodiment and Movement

In most lucid dreams, we are embodied: we have a body with which we explore the dream. This body is a mental projection, of course, just like everything else in the lucid dream. In an OBE, however, we may not have a body at all. We may be just a point of awareness dislocated from our physical body. This allows us to look at our body while we are out of it.

Everybody's experience will be unique, but for me, in a typical Locale I OBE I am a disembodied point of awareness or a transparent energy form which has separated from my physical body at the boundary of sleep and is then able to move through waking reality (or what seems to be waking reality) with a sense of friction, as if I have some sort of energetic mass that is interfering with the energy fields of that reality. Movement in a lucid dream

---

* It may seem that entry into an OBE from the lucid dream state is the best argument *against* OBEs being distinct from lucid dreams, but in fact this technique can be a great way to cross-reference the many differences between the two phenomena.

is usually smooth and easy to dictate whereas movement in an OBE 'will often be accompanied by intense vibration and energy disturbance'.[26] Whichever way you cut it, that's definitely not an experience found commonly in lucid dreaming.

Estimation of Time

In lucid dreams, time is relative to waking time (laboratory studies have found that a ten-minute lucid dream feels as though it has taken ten minutes) but in the OBE state, time is very different. What may feel like a four-hour OBE can turn out to have lasted only 20 minutes. This is a subtle but profound difference between the two.

Malleability

One of the easiest ways to tell if you are in an OBE or a lucid dream is to check the malleability of the environment: can you change things at will? If you can then you are probably in a lucid dream. In a lucid dream you can change aspects of the dreamscape because you are inside your personal mindstream, but in an OBE it is much more difficult to change things, because you are not in your personal mindstream, you're in a shared one.

In lucid dreams, the dreamscape is relative to expectation, but in an OBE, the 'expectation effect' is out of the window because it is not our mental expectations that are creating the environment.

As you can see, there are many different ways to tell the difference between an OBE and a lucid dream, but the easiest way to get to grips with these differences is to spend as much time as we can in these states. I still believe that there are some people who are mistakenly labelling pre-lucid dreams and false awakenings as OBEs, but I now know beyond all doubt that through true OBE experience you *can* intentionally leave your personal mindstream and the limitations of your own head.

THE TIBETAN BUDDHIST VIEW ON OBEs

In Tibetan Buddhism, both lucid dreaming and OBE work are found within the dream yoga practices and can be learned by practitioners who are grounded in meditation and ready to engage the practices. My teacher Lama Yeshe Rinpoche once described the difference between the two phenomena in very simple terms: 'Lucid dreaming? In your head. But, also, you can go out of your head!'

Those of you who are typically sceptical Buddhists, please relax those pursed lips and furrowed brows at this point, for it should be noted that the practice of separating the subtle energy body from the gross corporeal body has a long tradition in Tibetan Buddhism.* In fact even the wonderfully solid Akong Rinpoche once told me, 'Learning astral projection will be of benefit in the *bardo* state because that separation of the body and mind is exactly what happens in the after-death *bardo*. If you can learn the basics of this then, yes, that will be useful.'[27]

I should add that the separation of the subtle energy body from the gross physical body, which we find in some advanced Tibetan Buddhist meditations, is only ever taught within the safety of a retreat environment and under the guidance of a qualified master, unlike some of the new-agey 'OBE weekends' that we find offered in the West. Having an OBE can be an incredibly intense experience and so from a Buddhist point of view it is advised that you only engage the practice once you are well grounded in mindfulness and compassion training.

---

* Mindrolling Rinpoche, the renowned Tibetan lama who died in 2008, spent the last few years of his life in an almost constant state of lucid dreaming and astral projection, often practising dream yoga all day, projecting out of his body and interacting with waking reality.

OBEs AND LUCID DREAMS FOR SPIRITUAL GROWTH

So, if OBEs allow us to leave our personal mindstream and the limitations of our own head, is lucid dreaming just a stepping stone towards the more advanced practice of astral projection?

I don't think so. When we lucid dream, we are inside our own head, a place where we can work directly with our own personal psychology, a laboratory for enlightened action in which we can reprogramme our negative habitual tendencies for the benefit of both ourselves and all beings, creating new patterns of positive mind states which will profoundly affect the way we think and act. Lucid dreaming makes us kinder, wiser and more awake.

Similarly, OBEs are amazing tools for growth and a brilliant skill to foster alongside our lucid dreaming practice. They allow us to engage time in a much more flexible way, offering us the potential to experience what feels like hours of out-of-body exploration in a matter of minutes, and they allow us to communicate with energy systems and consciousnesses outside our own head. The big selling point of the OBE experience is that it profoundly shifts our view on reality, even more so than lucid dreaming, because it shows us that we are not limited to our own body and that we have the same quantum potentiality as the atoms that make up that body.

But without pure motivation and skilful application, all of this potential can end up being no more than a head trip – a head trip outside your own head.

When we have an OBE I don't believe that we are travelling to another physical dimension, but I do believe that we are travelling to another mental dimension, which, although it may seem to be separate from us, is in fact still within the realm of the larger universal mind that both encompasses and lies beyond the subjective limitations of our personal mind.

In fact, the name 'OBE' is quite misleading, because it implies that our consciousness is located somewhere in our body and so when we go beyond our personal mind we have gone 'out of our body', whereas our mind and sense of self were never confined to our body in the first place. Perhaps these experiences should be called 'into mind' rather than 'out of body'?

Neuro-anthropologist Charles Laughlin, PhD, says that the fundamental folly comes from the fact that many OBEers believe that 'they are floating "out there" rather than "in here" between their ears'.[28] Both Buddhism and quantum physics seem to side with Dr Laughlin on this one, because there is no reality that is not dependent, at least in part, on the consciousness that resides between our ears.

Charlie says

'Whether we are in our mind or out of our body, my advice is this: don't set up a duality within your spiritual practice. Mistaken duality has got us into enough trouble in the waking state already without us slipping into the same trap in our spiritual practice. However dualistic and separate the alternate dimensions that you visit in an OBE may seem, they are not separate, they are all part of you, and part of your mind in exactly the same way that waking reality is, too.'

Beyond Lucidity

*'You take the blue pill – the story ends, you wake up in
your bed and believe whatever you want to believe.
You take the red pill – you stay in Wonderland and I
show you how deep the rabbit-hole goes.'*
MORPHEUS, *THE MATRIX*

Lucid dreaming takes us beyond mere projection and into
aspects of mind that are in the frontier land of consciousness.
Once we decide to 'take the red pill' of lucidity, we start to see
'how deep the rabbit-hole goes' as we begin a journey which
may profoundly reconfigure not only our perception of our
dreams, but our perception of our waking life, too.

In this chapter let's ride into frontier land and explore the
germination of ideas that will challenge our accepted modes
of experience and call into question the very nature of waking
reality. Let's explore how to wake up from the waking dream and
live our life with lucidity as co-creators of the dream of being.

ONENESS: THE INTERCONNECTED NATURE OF REALITY

'See through the illusion of separateness and recognize that we are all one... Knowing that you are one with all, you will find yourself in love with all and you will fall in love with living.'[1]
GNOSTIC CHRISTIAN WISDOM

Many of the great spiritual traditions tell us that contrary to how we may feel, we are actually 'one with everything', interconnected with all, beyond any notion of separateness. This idea is usually referred to as 'Oneness'.

The key motivation for moving towards Oneness is based on the notion that separateness separates us, whereas oneness brings us together, with love, in love. Sounds simple, right? It's a lovely idea and a concept that's easy to understand theoretically, but in practice it can be very hard to see how the 'me, my, I', so distinctly different from 'you', and from the trees and buildings and animals that make up our reality, could ever *not* be separate.

There is, however, a direct way in which to make the theoretical understanding of Oneness experiential: lucid dreaming. Once lucid, we can actually experience the interconnected Oneness that we have heard about because in a lucid dream we are at one with all things. We are the trees, we are the leaves on the trees, we are the wind that blows through the leaves on the trees. Everything is us and we are everything. And as we enter into the experience of being one with everything, we know that we are dreaming the dream and everything in it into existence. Everything in the dream is part of the projection of our own mind – everything that seems so absolutely real and yet is so absolutely illusory. All aspects of the dream are within our own psyche and so there is no 'us and them', no duality, no separateness, just Oneness.

But it's still just a dream, right? Yes, of course, but once we wake up from a lucid dream in which we've experienced this sense of Oneness, we'll never look at waking reality in quite the same way again. Seeing our inherent Oneness is the beginning of real compassion, because it allows us to reach beyond separation and selfishness.

In a lucid dream, the trees and the people and the buildings look and feel so undeniably separate from us and yet we know that they're not separate because they are all part of our own mind. This knowledge leaves an indelible trace on our waking consciousness that allows us at least to question (and at most directly challenge) the very nature of a waking reality that looks and feels just as separate as the dream did. Lucid dreaming opens us up to the possibility of being one with all things.

> **Charlie says**
>
> 'In Part I we explored the Buddhist concept of Emptiness, and although it's easy to say that Emptiness and Oneness are the same thing, it's not quite that simple. Although, as my teacher says, to be empty of a separate identity means to be one with everything in the cosmos, the interconnected nature of Oneness and the illusory nature of Emptiness are quite different concepts and should not be confused.'

Quantum Dreaming

Through quantum physics we now understand that the objective world is almost as much a fantasy as our dreams. Separateness is an illusion, Oneness is reality – not only in our dreams but in the waking world, too. This is not conjecture, this is fact.

'Quantum physics reveals the basic oneness of the universe'[2] because it shows us that everything is interconnected beyond all notions of separateness just as it is in a lucid dream. Quantum physics has shattered the views of classical physics, which placed us as passive observers in a materialistic universe, because it has proved that we are integrally connected with everything in the entire cosmos.* But how does this actually work?

We now know that an atom only appears in a particular place if we measure it. This means that it is spread out all over the place until a conscious observer decides to look at it. This in turn shows us that the actual act of observation creates the whole universe. So, quantum physics tells us that physical reality is in large part an illusion that our consciousness conjures into existence.

If we tap our fingers on a table, for example, it seems solid, and yet it isn't solid, because it is made of atoms, and atoms aren't solid, they are 99.9999999999 per cent empty space. So, what creates the feeling of solidity? 'Our minds!' shout the pseudo-science crowd. Well, they're right in part, but it's not quite that simple. Apart from that crucial 0.00000001 per cent that actually does exist, it is the electromagnetic repulsion between the electrons in your fingers and those in the desk that stops your fingers passing through it. It is, however, our mind that interprets these electrostatic forces picked up by the pressure sensors in our fingers as the 'feeling of solidity'.**

It has been said that scientific materialism works on the belief that 'there is one indivisible material reality that is universally consistent. Scientists proposing this view believe in a world that can be seen as it actually is: separate from ourselves, out there, a world that can be experienced in exactly the same way no

---

* Although quantum theory in the West is presented as a new idea, in his book *You Are Here*, Christopher Potter believes it was first explored as far back as the 1700s, when Bishop Berkeley asked if an unobserved tree could be said to exist.

** Senior lecturer in chemical physics Dr Alan Taylor told me that 'the atoms are held together by electrostatic force and the quantum mechanical phenomenon of bonding. When you push against this electron distribution, it exerts an equal and opposite force back.'

matter where we are in it.'[3] However, as the Nobel physicist Werner Heisenberg said, 'The ontology of materialism rests upon the illusion that the kind of existence, the direct "actuality" of the world around us, can be extrapolated into the atomic range. This extrapolation is, however, impossible.'[4]

What does this mean? Briefly, it means that the world of materialistic relativity has now been proven to be largely an illusion. Modern scientific breakthroughs now show us that everything is in an interconnected state of oneness and affected by consciousness, just as in a lucid dream. This may come as a shocking truth but, as Nobel Prize-winning physicist Niels Bohr said, 'Those who are not shocked when they first come across quantum theory cannot possibly have understood it.'[5]

Through lucid dreaming we are developing the habit of recognition and the capacity to directly challenge the illusion of dualistic materialism. This is because once we're lucid, we wake up to the fact that what we previously accepted as reality is actually just a mirage, empty of inherent existence, and, more importantly, we become aware that our consciousness, the observer, is creating this dream reality, just as it creates our waking reality.

So, lucid dreaming trains us to awaken to the quantum interconnectivity of life. It trains us to recognize the Oneness of waking reality. It trains us for the awakening of enlightenment. It has been said that once enlightened, we 'awaken from the dream of being a separate "me" to being the universal reality'[6] and that we wake up to the fact that however dualistic reality seems, there is in fact no 'I' and 'other'. There is no separateness, no division. We are the universal reality of all things, in waking life just as in a lucid dream.

DREAMING OUR REALITY INTO EXISTENCE?

Those who dream by night wake in the day to find that it was vanity: but the dreamers of the day are dangerous men, for they act out their dreams with open eyes, to make it possible.
T. E. LAWRENCE

If quantum physics shows us that through the act of observation our consciousness creates our reality, then perhaps the quality and intent of our consciousness can affect the creation of that reality?

With so much of experiential reality being governed by our mental outlook, habitual tendencies and personal projection, it doesn't take much to see that in many ways we really are the co-creators of our own reality. 'Two men look out of prison bars, one sees mud, the other sees stars', as the old saying goes. We are constantly projecting, and this kind of psychological projection is one of the most dominant forces of the human mind – and one that can be transformed into a powerful force of creation.

This concept forms the basis of the newly rejuvenated trend for 'manifestation'. We are told by some new age 'gurus' that if we powerfully visualize getting that new car and set our intent strongly enough then we will manifest a new car – or boob job , or pay rise, or a host of other unfortunately samsarically focused goals. These kinds of manifestation practices are actually based on sound spiritual principles that have been unfortunately diluted and repackaged for modern-day consumers. I believe that their weakness lies in a two-fold misinterpretation of how manifestation works. They misinterpret 'beneficial motivation' as 'ego motivation' and mistake 'action' for 'desire'.

It takes much more than just making a 'vision board' and really desiring to have lots of money for these things to actually manifest. Just as our level of influence over a lucid dream is only ever that of a co-creator, working alongside the unconscious mind and dependent on our beneficial motivation, so our level of influence over waking life is held within the constraints of the larger universal consciousness. And, vitally, our current experience of waking reality is dictated in large part by the results of our actions, our karma. That's the real secret.

Karma

Some people don't believe in the hands of fate or of a creator God calling the shots on a prearranged future. Instead they believe that they are the masters of their own destiny; they believe in something called karma. Karma is one of the most misunderstood tenets of Eastern spirituality, but one of the most important to understand in view of dreaming your reality into existence.

Within Buddhism, 'karma does not mean punishment. It is the law of cause and effect. If you want to grow a cabbage then you plant a cabbage seed (cause) and a cabbage grows (effect).'[7] If you plant an acorn hoping for a cabbage, you will end up disappointed, because you will grow an oak tree instead. You have not been *punished* – you are simply experiencing the result of planting a certain seed.

Karma means that we are the masters of our own destiny, because we create our future in the present moment through the seeds we choose to plant. If we want to be happy in the future, we need to plant the seeds of happiness (being kind and helping others). These seeds will then sprout in the form of happiness and beneficial circumstances.

Our karma is of course linked to everybody else's karma, too. The Buddhist nun Pema Chödron says that because everything is karmically interconnected, 'If you hurt another person, you hurt yourself, and if you hurt yourself, you are hurting another person… We are not in this alone. We are all in this together.'[8]

Our actions count. This is how karma forms the basis not only of our future happiness but also that of those around us. Karma is the opposite of fate: it means that the future is in our hands because what we do now creates our future.[9]

The word *karma* means 'action' and so with every action of our body, speech and mind we are creating our future reality. So, within us lies the potential to be whatever we choose. By understanding karma we really can dream our reality into existence, but if we ignore it we risk our dream becoming a nightmare.

In a lucid dream we are literally dreaming our experiential reality into being because we are influencing and co-creating the dream with our conscious intent. But however skilled we become at this in our dreams, in the waking state we have our karma to deal with, too. This means that fervently desiring money or wishing really hard for a new car without engaging any beneficial action (karma), which might lead to the manifestation of that money or new car, is unlikely to have much effect.

The Placebo Effect

A more everyday example of how we dream our reality into existence is through the placebo effect, which Professor Richard Wiseman from the University of Hertfordshire says has been shown to account for a staggering 60–90 per cent of the effectiveness of some medical drugs.[10]

Sounds unbelievable? Let's hear from a man who has made it his life's work to study things beyond belief. The sceptic epidemiologist Dr Ben Goldacre is passionate about dispelling health myths created by the dissemination of misleading scientific data. Yet even someone like Dr Goldacre believes that the placebo effect is one of the most fascinating concepts in the whole of medicine and concludes that for some ailments, 'two sugar pills a day is the most effective treatment available. Two sugar pills a day beats one sugar pill a day. And that's an outrageous and ridiculous finding, but it's true. It's all about our beliefs and expectations.'[11] Our mind really does create our experience of waking reality, just as it does in our dreams.

A placebo effect study cited by Professor Richard Wiseman has proved that we can affect the way we think, interact with the world and physically behave based purely on our mental perception and illusory input.

Researchers got together a group of students and after assessing their current cognitive ability randomly assigned them to two groups, red and blue. Both groups were then asked to go into a room where there was a free bar and to order and drink as many beverages as they liked. Although the students didn't know it, only one of the groups, the red group, was actually served alcoholic drinks over the course of the experiment. The blue group was served drinks that tasted and smelled identical to alcoholic drinks but were actually alcohol-free.

Throughout the evening, students of both groups were regularly tested for cognitive ability and the results showed that the students who were part of the blue group, and therefore had not ingested a single drop of alcohol, became just as drunk as those who actually had. They displayed signs not only of physical inebriation, lack of balance and coordination, but signs of mental inebriation, too. They had significant memory impairment and their minds had entered into a drunken state of consciousness. Just believing that they had been drinking alcohol 'was enough to convince their brains and bodies to behave in a drunk way'.[12]

What this study shows is that our mental outlook and beliefs about ourselves affect our body and mind, which in turn do their best to make these beliefs a reality, just as when we dream.

The Shared Dream

Albert Einstein once asked Niels Bohr, 'Do you really believe that the moon is not there when nobody looks at it?' To that Bohr replied, 'Can you prove to me the opposite: that the moon is still there when nobody looks?' Their interaction makes me wonder: are we really seeing the same reality as everybody else?

The answer is no. The information coming in from our eyes, through the thalamus and into the back of the brain only makes up 10 per cent of the overall information that we use to see.[13] The other 90 per cent comes from other parts of the brain and not from 'out there' at all. This means that what we see through our eyes is only one tenth of reality and so 'rather than seeing what is physically present, the way we see the world is mostly based upon our prediction of the world'.[14]

People say 'I'll believe it when I see it!' but it seems that in fact we'll see it when we believe it, because, as neuroscientist Dr Beau Lotto says, 'Seeing is literally believing. We see what we believe.'[15] When the world becomes too familiar, our brain reverts to a kind of 'automatic pilot' which stops seeing what is right in front of our eyes, meaning that for much of the time we're not seeing the exact same world as everybody else.

It seems that reality is based upon our interaction with it and that our consciousness co-creates our experience of the world. Could lucid dream training help us to learn how to play a part in this creation? The dream yogis seem to think so. The late Traleg Rinpoche said that 'every time we change our dreams we increase our capacity to change our conscious experience while we are awake'[16] and that by training our capacity to direct a lucid dream we are enhancing our ability to direct the dream of waking reality. This is how lucid dreaming leads to lucid living.

LUCID LIVING

Imagine the bliss of becoming lucid at all times, perceiving all things as luminous displays of the deepest dimension of our own awareness. This is the truth that sets us free.
B. ALAN WALLACE

For thousands of years Buddhism has proffered that although we believe that we are awake, our waking lives are actually spent sleepwalking through a dreamlike illusion that we mistake for absolute reality. As we learned earlier, scientists and quantum physicists now agree that what we perceive to be a solid, permanent reality is actually more like a shared projection. With only 0.00000000001 per cent of perceived form being existent, we partially project mind into form, just as we do in our dreams.

In waking life, however, most of us are still not aware that the majority of reality is a dreamlike illusion and so we feel separate from and threatened by everything that we perceive to be not us. This perceived threat leads to fear and we become afraid of 'the other' and barricade ourselves in against the shock of mistaken dualism. In a lucid dream, however, we become aware that we are dreaming and 'wake up' to the illusion that what we once thought to be a solid, permanently existing reality is actually just a projection of our own mind. Once we have experienced this awakening, we begin to relax and enjoy the show a bit more in our waking life, because we are aware that it is not quite as solid and inflexible as we have been led to believe.

Every time we lucid dream we are experiencing a new perception of reality, one in which we are the co-creator, and the more we experience this, the more we may also perceive waking reality in a similar way. Each time we do this we are creating a habit of recognition. It is this habit of seeing through illusion that forms the crux of lucid living.

Lucid dreamers naturally begin to take charge of their waking life in much the same way as they do in their dreams. Empowered by the experiences of their lucid dreams, they strive consciously to direct and co-create their waking lives, too. They become more positive, proactive and discerningly optimistic in their waking interactions. They embrace the shadow elements of daily life fearlessly* and work through psychological blocks more creatively as they begin to take back the reins of their lives and live more lucidly.

Charlie says

'One of the first people I saw demonstrate lucid living in action was Robert Waggoner. We had a pint at a pub after one of his dream workshops and he wanted to get a black cab back to his hotel. We were in a residential area on a Sunday evening, so I told him that there was no chance of this happening, but he started going on about the interconnectedness of reality and that if we really expected to find a black cab, then we could "intend" one into existence. To be honest, I thought that was just the beer talking, but then suddenly we saw an empty black cab parked outside a house. As we looked at it, a man came out of the house and got into it. He was just starting his shift. Robert looked at me and said, "You see, Charlie, it's all about expectation!" '

How Does It Actually Work?

In a fully lucid dream we experience a boost of awareness that facilitates the realization that we are conscious within our own psyche. This extraordinary awareness reveals that what we thought was separate from us, outside us, apart from us, is in fact inside us and at one with us. Imagine if we could have a similar

---

* Once you've hugged a terrifying shadow monster or turned to face the recurring nightmare that has been haunting you for years, being brave enough to stand up to a bully just doesn't seem that scary any more!

realization in this dream of waking reality. Imagine if we could become lucid while we were awake…

We know that if we want to start having lucid dreams we need to engage three core principles: strong motivation, effective techniques and, most importantly, a shift in mental perspective which gives us the confidence to believe that lucidity is possible. Similarly, if we engage these three core principles while awake, we can learn to have moments of lucidity in the shared dream of waking life.

Why would we want to become lucid in waking life? Because once we are fully lucid and awake, our human potential is fully realized. In fact if we were to wake up completely from this dream, we would become a buddha: one who has woken up. Enlightenment is described as waking from the dream of being a separate entity to the realization that we are the universal reality of all things.

The more aware and lucid we can be in our daily life, the kinder we can be to ourselves and others. Kindness is the basis of lasting happiness and we all want to be happy, right? I once asked my teacher Lama Yeshe Rinpoche what the point of being more awake was and he replied with a sentence which I think encompasses the entire spiritual path: 'More awake, more aware. More aware, more kind. More kind: that's the whole point!'[17]

But surely we are awake already? If you are reading this sentence then you must be awake, right? Partially, yes, but just as there are multiple stages of sleep, so there are different stages of wakefulness. It seems strange that we use the word 'awake' to describe everything from pre-sleep drowsiness to post-caffeine alertness. Our entire daily experience is called 'awake' and yet think how it fluctuates. Even when we claim to be awake, Harvard research has shown that most of us are unaware, on autopilot or not in the present moment for 47 per cent of our waking life.[18] We may appear to be awake, but we are definitely not fully lucid much of the time.

How Can We Live More Lucidly?

I'm not living lucidly every day of my life, just as I'm not lucid dreaming every night of my life. But as with lucid dreaming, which I can do whenever I apply the techniques and put in the effort, I've learned how to have flashes of lucidity in waking life. Here are a few of the techniques that help us to live a bit more lucidly.

Meditation

Meditation is one of the original methods for lucid living. It has been found cross-culturally since the Akashic records began. It may seem a rather paradoxical method: we think that we will keep ourselves awake by constantly doing things, but actually one of the best ways to wake ourselves up is to do nothing – the intentional and very active nothing of mindfulness meditation.

Meditation brings us into direct contact with our inner environment and through this we come to know ourselves better and so become better equipped to know when we are on autopilot and when we are truly awake. Meditation is also a form of mind training in which we make our mind stronger, more flexible and healthier. Just as it's impossible to get fit without doing any exercise, so it's impossible to wake up and live lucidly without exercising our mind.

Mind training is like going to the mind gym; it's about flexing the muscles of our mind to give ourselves the strength to become lucid. Researchers at Harvard, Yale, and MIT have found conclusive evidence that regular periods of meditation can actually alter the physical structure of our brain in favour of clarity and lucid awareness.[19] There is no greater tool on our path to lucid living than meditation and I implore you to engage some sort of regular meditation practice if you can.*

---

* Check out Chapter 6 if you need a reminder of how to practise mindfulness meditation.

Life Signs

As we know, dream signs are any aspect of the dream experience that can be used to indicate that we are dreaming. They are triggers that help us become lucid within the dream, but there are also triggers in waking life that can help us become more lucid. I call these 'life signs'.

A life sign is any aspect of our waking experience that reveals the dreamlike nature of reality and helps to wake us from our slumber. Synchronicities, coincidences and flashes of intuition are all potential life signs. Anytime you experience one of these things, be sure to acknowledge it and allow it to wake you up. This is very similar to the Columbo Method that we learned earlier.

The most powerful way to lucid living is to regard waking life as a little bit more dreamlike. Intentionally looking out for life signs will help this shift of perception to take place. This forms the foundation of a Tibetan Buddhist practice called Illusory Body yoga, which is used in conjunction with dream yoga to help the practitioner realize the dreamlike nature of reality.

Be careful not to turn all this into some sort of ego trip, though. Everybody is part of the same dream, so you are no more the central protagonist than anybody else. Having said that, don't be blasé or try to act cool whenever something dreamlike happens. Instead, acknowledge it and be thankful for the opportunity for lucidity.

Charlie says

'English people like myself seem to be the worst at recognizing life signs. If a genie were to pop out of a bottle of beer in an English pub, the most that you'd get from the punters would be a raised eyebrow! But lucid living requires us to notice life signs and allow them to raise our level of awareness, not ignore them out of embarrassment.'

Think about Death More

Buddhist scholar Stephen Batchelor says that one of the paradoxes of the human condition is that 'by meditating on death we become more conscious of life'.[20] In fact there is no more visceral way to wake up to life than by thinking about death.

Death is a shared commonality of human experience and yet we hardly ever talk about it, at least not in the West. We seldom discuss it or plan for it or talk about how we would like it to happen. It's as if we think it won't happen at all and yet we *will* all die. Definitely.

Charlie says

'Our egoic sense of self dupes us into thinking that if we contemplate death or even mention its name we will somehow hasten its arrival or jinx ourselves. This is absolute rubbish! Our ego tells us this to maintain its stranglehold over our higher self, and every time we give in to the fear, we feed it and so its power over us increases. The "me, my, I" hates contemplating death because it fears the boost of awareness and lucidity to which that contemplation will lead.'

Contemplating death wakes us up to our own potentiality but also to our limitations of time. Most people have 100 years max. to live their life and to offer something of value to the human story. The great master Dilgo Khyentse Rinpoche once said, 'On the day that you were born, you began to die. Do not waste a single moment more!'[21] This sounds extreme, but he knew that mortality awareness helps us to be more motivated, compassionate and lucid.

Contemplating death is a great way to live more lucidly, so I ask you to take a few minutes now to ask yourself this: if you were to die one week from now, would you be able to die at peace with the world? Take time to really contemplate that question, make notes if you like and then see what actions you might be able to engage in to make it possible. Don't wait till you're on your deathbed to make your peace, do it this week while you still have time.

Act Lucid

I have found that as their practice matures, many lucid dreaming practitioners report that three primary mental attitudes arise within their lucid dreams. These are acceptance, friendliness and kindness.

Acceptance arises from the realization that everything we are seeing, experiencing and interacting with is a projection of our mind and an expression of our own potentiality. Once we have accepted this, we find that friendliness towards everything in the dream arises naturally, because all of it is a part of us. With this friendliness comes a feeling of kindness, as we treat everything in the dream with the kindness with which we would treat ourselves.

> **Charlie says**
>
> 'A few years ago, acceptance, friendliness and kindness started to manifest in my own lucid dreams more and more. I remember one lucid dream in particular in which these three mental attitudes showed themselves most obviously. I found myself fully lucid, hugging a chair and feeling as connected to that chair as I would to a close friend!' (For a full description of this dream, see Dream 16, page 259.)

If in waking life we truly believed that everything we were seeing, experiencing and interacting with was part of us, just as in a lucid dream, we would find that acceptance, friendliness and kindness arose spontaneously. Unfortunately, this is dependent upon us living lucidly enough to believe it in the first place, which in my experience is easier said than done. But if acceptance, friendliness and kindness arise *from* lucidity in our dreams, perhaps they can *lead to* lucidity in our waking life?

They can and they do. By replicating the mental attitudes of a lucid dream in the waking state, we can create the conditions needed to become lucid in everyday life. To become lucid in life, we just need to start acting lucidly!

Let's Do It!

Act with acceptance: in this context, 'acceptance' means unconditional love towards ourselves and towards all situations in which we find ourselves, however unpleasant they may seem. It does *not* mean approval or endorsement of negative mind states or situations. It is, however, a prerequisite to actively engaging with negative situations and doing something about them.

If we truly accept not only our present moment but also that we are interconnected with every single other being in the universe, we will definitely start to live with more love and lucidity.

Act with friendliness: to live lucidly is to approach all situations, good and bad, with unconditional friendliness – that's friendliness towards ourselves, towards others, towards negative emotions, towards change and pain. That is the path to lucid living.

Living lucidly is actually impossible without a mental attitude of unconditional friendliness. Why? Because duality is based upon unfriendliness and selfishness. Every time we believe that we are more important than everyone else, we further cement the grasp that duality has over us. But the moment that we see others as equally important or even more important than ourselves (shock horror!) we seem to short-circuit the dreamy dualism of waking life and become more lucid within it.

Act with kindness: be kind to everything in this life because, just as in a lucid dream, everything is connected to you. Every time we are unkind to someone we are further strengthening the non-lucid belief that we are separate from them. You know that warm feeling after being kind to someone or really helping another person? I believe that warmth is the somatic manifestation of lucidity.

Charlie says

'By cultivating acceptance, friendliness and kindness, we stand a far greater chance of living lucidly. Why? Because we are recreating the dominant mind states of fully lucid dreaming while we are awake! It's such a simple idea, but I urge you to try it – it really does help to wake you up.'

We can all live with a little more lucidity, but we have to work at it, just as we do with lucid dreaming. Sometimes we might have flashes of spontaneous lucidity in our life, just as we may have spontaneous lucid dreams, but for the most part we need to plan for lucidity. This is fine, of course, but as one Tibetan master commented, 'You like plans, so make your plan, but then put it in your back pocket and live your life in the present moment. Your plan will always be there if you need it.'[22]

Those who practise lucid living aren't procrastinators, they're doers. So be wise and mindful and don't rush into anything, but at the same time don't get stuck at the planning stage; go out and make things happen. Show the dream that you are ready to co-create it – dance with karma and dream your destiny into existence.

Awakening within the Dream

'To awaken within the dream is our purpose now. When we are awake within the dream, the ego-created earth-drama comes to an end and a more benign and wondrous dream arises.'
ECKHART TOLLE, *A NEW EARTH*

When I was 13, I was sent to an ex-military boarding school. It was a fruitless but compassionate attempt by my parents to get me back onto the rails of discipline. It was there that I not only became interested in philosophy and Buddhism but also met one of the most curiously intelligent people I had ever come across. He was a wonderfully 'old school' literature master called Dr Fox and he once told me a story I would never forget – a story about impossibility.

One day when he was a child, sitting at the breakfast table, his mother asked his father for a cigarette. His father reached into his breast pocket, pulled a cigarette from its packet and casually threw it at the breakfast table. It landed not on its side or rolling across the table, but in a perfectly upright position. Dr Fox said that from that day onwards, he knew that nothing was impossible.

That story left an indelible mark on my mind – far more so than the seemingly impossible stories of levitating lamas and clairvoyant gurus that I have heard of since. I believe we should be careful before we brand something 'impossible'. It's a lazy label most often used by cynics and sceptics who seem to be the voice of reason – until we discover as E. E. Barnard did that there *is* more than one galaxy in our universe and the dream state *can* be experienced consciously.

Lucid dreaming is just one former 'impossibility', which in turn opens the door to further seemingly incredible notions. Whether it's communication with our higher self, lucidly prophesied events or insights into the dreamlike nature of waking reality, at some point in our lucidity training we will be challenged to re-evaluate the boundaries of what is possible. It is how we respond to that challenge that counts, because our potential awakening may be dependent upon it.

The central metaphor within Buddhism is that of awakening from a dream. The word *Buddha* actually means 'awakened one' and it's said the only difference between us and a fully enlightened buddha is that they have woken up. Woken up from what? From the illusion of separateness, just as we do in a lucid dream.

It's said that sometime after his enlightenment under the bodhi tree, the Buddha was travelling along the road when he encountered a priest walking towards him. This man was astonished by the Buddha's radiating energy and asked him: 'Are you a god?'

The Buddha replied, 'No.'

'Are you an angel?'

The Buddha again replied, 'No.'

'Are you a spirit then?'

The Buddha replied, 'No.'

The priest tried a fourth time, asking, 'Are you a man?'

Again the Buddha replied, 'No.'

Finally the priest asked, 'Well, what are you then?'

The Buddha replied, 'I am awake.'

The Buddha was neither a god nor an angel nor a spirit; he was a human being who had woken up into a state beyond the limitations of the dualistic self and had made the impossible possible by becoming fully lucid in all states of day and night.

Through lucid dreaming we can get a taste of this awakening as we experience the extraordinary awareness that we are both within the illusion of the dream while simultaneously dreaming everything in the dream into existence. This experience leads to direct insight into the nature of the illusion that binds us to *samsara*. This experience can wake us up.

ONWARDS INTO THE DREAM

If you sleep, you dream, and if you dream, you can lucid dream. Whether you sleep in the park or the palace, lucid dreaming is available to you. It is your birthright. Unrestricted by censorship or state control, limited only by the relationship with your own inner state, lucid dreaming is a taste of true freedom.

If properly cultivated, lucidity training may become one of the greatest advancements in psychological self-development that the 21st century has ever seen. Its potential is huge and yet at present we are barely scratching the surface. I believe that lucid dreaming, (or at least awareness of how sleep and dream can be used for psycho-spiritual development), could become part of children's education in much the same way as mindfulness is being introduced into some British schools today. I envisage a time when we may have 'lucid dream therapists' who will use the medium of the lucid dream to help their clients commune with aspects of their unconscious. Just as we might have a 4 p.m. appointment with our hypnotherapist, so we might have a

4 a.m. appointment with our lucid dreaming therapist, who will be ready to guide us into sleep and advise on what to do in our next lucid dream.

The parallels between hypnosis and lucid dreaming being accepted as a verified therapeutic treatment are quite relevant. The psychological benefits of hypnosis were known about for hundreds of years, but it wasn't until the 1950s that the American and British Medical Associations approved hypnotherapy as an orthodox treatment. It is also likely to take time for the therapeutic benefits of lucid dreaming to be validated by Western medical science, but eventually it will happen. When it does, as a reader of this book you will be able to count yourself as a frontier explorer, a pioneer who was willing to engage the magical potential of lucidity before the majority. And not just the wider majority but even the majority of spiritual seekers, too, because as Lama Yeshe Rinpoche says, 'In the West, most people, even Buddhists, have not yet fully understood the real potential of lucid dreaming. But once people know how important this is, everyone will practise it!'[1]

Lucid dreaming is a movement, and you are now part of it. If there ever comes a time when a bizarre occurrence on a London tube train is met with a carriage full of people flipping their hands as a reality check, or a time when 'lucid dreaming' is a household term, we will know that this movement has made it into the mindstream of the mainstream. And I want it to become mainstream. It's not the fashionable preserve of some spiritual élite, it's one of the most accessible mind-training methods in existence, and it requires nothing more than sleep to practise it. Don't keep lucid dreaming to yourself – share it with others and you will share a gift more precious than any object, because you will share a potential that, if realized, may change their lives forever.

The Buddhist master Dilgo Khyentse Rinpoche once said, 'The outer universe – the earth, stones, mountains, rocks, and cliffs – seems to be permanent and stable, like the city built of concrete. In fact, there is nothing solid to it at all; it is nothing but a city of dreams.' Into this city of dreams we are born over and over again, unaware of the matrix of illusion that creates it. Lucid dreaming shows us how to make friends with illusion while we sleep so that we can be free from illusion while we're awake.

To lucid dream is to peep behind the magician's curtain. This doesn't spoil the magic, though. Once we see how the illusion works, it ceases to have power over us. We still enjoy the show, but we watch less with awe and more with laughter. Through lucid dreaming we learn how to wake up and smile at the magic. So let us move onwards together, as dreamers in the same dream, onto a path of awakening...

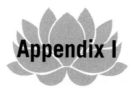

Appendix I

A Selection of Lucid Dreams

The following dreams, all referenced in Chapter 8, are taken directly from my own dream diaries. They have been transcribed exactly as written, but I have taken the liberty of editing out any insignificant or boring bits.

The 'prep before bed' parts are lists of the techniques, causes and conditions that may have led to that particular lucid dream. It's a good habit to get into making these lists, because it allows you to see any patterns that emerge and to analyse which techniques work best for you.

Dream I: Short Lucid Dancing Dream
18 May 2012

I dreamed that I was at the Hippodrome nightclub with Ed and the rest of the crew. A girl at the bar was asking for a drink in a very strange way and I thought that I might be dreaming. I glanced over at Ed and saw that he was dancing funnily and as he danced he looked at me and said, 'It's all a dream!' I instantly did a hand reality check and realized that I was dreaming.

I then joined Ed on the dance floor next to the bar and began dancing really stupidly, secure in the knowledge that there could be no embarrassment or ego in a club populated by my own psyche! It felt so liberating to dance without ego! The dream characters surrounding the dance floor initially sneered at my silly dancing, but once I looked back at them with confidence and acceptance, their faces soon changed.

To dance inside my own mind without any need to look cool or dance well felt so liberating! It felt so good to move my body in childlike ways and to dance like a fool. There was wisdom in its foolishness. The dance was like an offering of naïvety and surrender. I felt that I had found my dancer.

Dream 2: Career Path Lucidity
27 August 2010

After weeks of doubt over whether I was qualified to teach, I dreamed that I was watching a big house fill up with water and burst under the pressure. I watched the doors and windows explode outwards, gushing water out and forming a tsunami that rushed out of the house onto the street on which I stood! After an initial flash of fear I thought to myself, I reckon I can surf this wave – I'm gonna be alright! and I bodysurfed the tsunami as it swept me off my feet.

The fear seemed to boost my awareness and I soon became fully lucid. I realized within the dream that the house bursting under pressure was symbolic of the doubt that I had been feeling recently. So then I thought that this would be the perfect opportunity to ask my higher self/unconscious mind for some advice about this.

After a couple of reality checks to solidify the lucidity, I called out to the sky, 'How can I be of most benefit? Should I do the lucid dreaming or should I do Throwdown [the hip-hop group that I used to run]?'

In an instant the entire dreamscape dissolved from the suburban street into a drinks party in the living room of a small house. The room was full of people standing around chatting and I realized beyond doubt that each person in the room was an aspect of my own psyche who would have an answer to my question.

I spotted a man in white robes who looked like a cross between a Buddhist monk and a vicar (a personification of my spiritual side?) and I went up to him and asked, 'What should I do with my life? Should I teach lucid dreaming or do Throwdown?'

He replied with great sincerity and clasped his hands in prayer, saying, 'Of course, you must do the lucid dream teaching. That is of most benefit.'

Then I saw a teenager standing in the corner of the room, knocking back shots (a personification of my hedonistic side?) and I went up to him and asked the same question. His reply was to offer me a shot of vodka and yell, 'Throwdown rocks, man!'

Still with full lucidity and chuckling to myself about how my unconscious was choosing to portray my wild side, I then went and asked a pretty neutral-looking woman and a 30-something man what they thought I should do with my life, and they both said that I should do the lucid dream teaching, too.

Satisfied that I had got a balanced opinion from these aspects of my own psyche, I walked out of the house and found myself on an urban street at dusk. Why hadn't I woken up yet? I usually wake up after I've been given the punchline/teaching.

As I walked away from the house, I was thinking about how supportive my unconscious had been. Then I suddenly felt the urge to turn round and look back at the house. I did and I saw all the dream characters that I had just been talking to huddled around the window watching me walk away. When they saw me turn round, they all started smiling and waving. It was so unexpected!

I felt as though my heart would burst with joy and I yelled out, 'Unconscious, subconscious, conscious mind, I love you all! Thank you so much for everything!'

Then the dream characters started calling out, 'Good luck, Charlie! We love you, too!'

I woke up because of the wetness of tears on my pillow. I was crying with happiness. Any doubt over what I should do with my life was gone. I felt an unshakable confidence and faith.

Dream 3: Meeting my Subconscious Mind
13 May 2009

This was one of those rare lucid dreams in which the healing is so deep that you can actually feel it physically the next day. A deep underlying happiness and contentment lasted for the entire day that followed and I'm not sure it has ever completely faded.

I was in a large open-plan office space which was in a basement. There were people milling about as if some sort of 'Ideal Home Show' exhibition had finished a few hours before. I heard a man telling his son, 'Make a living! You just need to make a living!' and I felt annoyed at him for giving his son such limiting advice. For some reason I decided to do some cartwheels around the space to show the boy how he could free his thinking. The movement seemed to tip me over into lucidity and I realized that I was dreaming.

After doing a hand reality check, I became fully lucid. I tried to remember the lucid dream plan I had made, but I couldn't seem to access my memory. Eventually, after a few seconds I remembered the plan: to meet my subconscious mind.

Instantly the dream plan became engaged, as all the dream characters disappeared. Just then a plain-looking woman in her early 30s appeared out of nowhere holding a clipboard. Instinctively

I knew that she was something to do with this dream plan, so I went up to her and said, 'Are you my subconscious?'

She replied, 'Yes, I am.'

I felt shocked – I hadn't actually been expecting her to say yes. I asked her again, 'So, you're my subconscious mind?'

Again she said in a matter of fact way, 'Yes, that's right.'

I was lost for words, but eventually I got my head together and said, 'Oh, OK. Great. Well… how am I?'

She replied, 'You're good. You're fine really.'

I then felt an overwhelming desire to confess to her and to apologize to her for all that I'd put us through. So I began admitting to all the bad things I'd done in my life and apologizing about all the people I'd wronged. There was no guilt, though – it felt good. It was an experience of real catharsis and once I'd finished the woman smiled and said, 'It's all right. I know you're working on that.' She was so accepting of me and not angry or judgemental.

It felt that there was nothing left to be said, so I hugged her and I woke up crying with happiness. Lying in my bed, I felt very different. Something had shifted.

Prep before Bed

Taught the MILD technique that evening and then practised MILD after 7:15 a.m. Wake-up.

Dream 4: 'What is the Essence of All Knowledge?'
9 May 2009

I dreamed that I was at a big theatre-type venue doing a gig with my old band. After the gig I was doing gravity-defying aerial acrobatics around the venue. The jumping up and down seemed to stimulate my lucid awareness [somatic sensation often leads to lucidity] and soon I was fully lucid.

I remembered my dream plan and put it into action. I called out to the dream: 'What is the essence of all knowledge?'

Instantly a huge game show-style computer screen manifested in front of me with the question written across it in big digital lettering. The letters were so big that I could read them easily without them blurring. Three dots appeared after the question mark, indicating that I was about to receive the answer.

I tried hard to keep my excitement under control, but it was really difficult! Then the answer finally manifested. The computer screen read: 'The essence of all knowledge is?... Obtainable through lucid dreaming'!

I literally laughed out loud within the dream as I thought, At least my unconscious has a sense of humour! Then I woke up.

Once awake, I opened to the possibility that maybe the answer wasn't such a joke after all. Maybe the essence of all knowledge is obtainable through lucid dreaming?

Prep before Bed
Listened to a Lama Surya Das audiobook while I fell asleep, plus I had a little bit of REM rebound from the night before. I did the FAC technique. Also, I went to sleep on a light stomach and had been thinking about how heartbreak can be good for lucid dreams.

Dream 5: Huge Lucid Dream with Walking through Walls and Entry into the Void!
22 April 2011

After two false awakenings I became fully lucid. My lucidity has been so slack recently that I really wanted to make this a nice long LD to really get back on track. I called out, 'Stabilize lucidity! The lucidity is deep and stable!' and my lucid awareness deepened.

The dreamscape was a big airy high-ceilinged shopping mall full of people walking around shopping. As I walked through the mall I decided to do some wall-walking. I went up to a dark granite stone wall which formed part of a shop front, reminded myself, I'm dreaming so I can stick my hand through this wall, then stuck my hand into it up to my elbow.

I took time to really experience how it felt. It was as if my arm was in a vat of partially solidified concrete. It was a thick viscous liquid rock and when I clasped at it I could feel the detail of the coarse grains of granite through my fingertips. I even managed to pull a handful of the liquid rock out of the wall, too. I watched as it collected like mercury in the palm of my hand and began to harden before my very eyes.

I then set the intention that the wall would now be solid and I tapped on it and it was kind of solid, like liquid with a hard film over it.

I looked around, saw another wall that formed part of a different shop and decided to run through it. I set the intention that on the other side of the wall I would find the dazzling darkness of the void. As I ran through the wall, I called out, 'Clear light now! For the benefit of all beings, clear light now!'

On the other side of the wall I found myself floating in the vast deep-space blackness of the void. From within the blackness huge archetypal images of golden light manifested. Snakes, dragons and ancient-looking creatures were traced in gold across the blackness. They began flicking up into my field of vision in very quick succession and it felt like some sort of download of information from the collective mind into my mind. It soon became too intense and I woke up.

Prep before Bed

Went to sleep after 20 minutes of meditation on reversed red Tibetan 'ah' in throat chakra. Then fell asleep sounding the 'ah' sound and offering prayers for lucidity. Fifteen minutes of meditation at shrine from 5 a.m. Woke again after LD at 6:45 a.m.

Dream 6: Ear-Infection Healing Dream

6 August 2012

I went surfing in New York and picked up a nasty ear infection that blocked my ear completely with wax – 'glue ear', they called it. I tried eardrops (and everything else I could think of), but they didn't seem to work, so I stopped using them. A few days later I became lucid and experienced my first direct physical manifestation of healing from within the lucid dream state.

Woke at about 4 a.m. after a very long healing lucid dream! Got lucid from the lights in the dream not working and hand reality checks. First I called out to all the dream characters, 'You are all aspects of my own psychology and I love you all!' Then I went over to a guy in a linen jacket and started touching the jacket, exploring how amazingly real it felt. I asked him what the material was and he said, 'Crosshatched brushed cotton.'

I said, 'What? I don't think I even know what that is.'

He replied, 'Maybe it's from your memory stores?'

Then I remembered my dream plan and engaged it: 'Heal my ear! Please, immune system, engage our healing power to heal me of my ear infection! Please help me to heal my glue ear! My ear is healed!'

Within the dream, I could actually hear and feel my ear being unblocked. It felt so realistic. I could hear the wax being broken up in my ear canal as if I had just put in eardrops! The sensation woke me up and I discovered that the dream had actually manifested a physical response! That's why it felt so realistic! Lying in my bed, wide awake, my ear was now unblocking and wax was streaming out of it. So gross, but so cool!

Dream 7: Exploring the Dreamscape and Befriending Shadow Aspects

28 April 2011

I dreamed that I was leaving a house when I saw a coach full of aggressors come roaring down the road towards me. In response to the fear, I became lucid.

Once lucid, I was in the grounds of a big school and my first thought was This is all just a projection of my mind! The lucidity wasn't actually that clear, so I boosted it by stating out loud: 'Stabilize lucidity!'

My dream plan was to explore the emptiness of the dream, so I started exploring the dreamscape by running my hands over the leaves of a plant in a nearby hedge. I could feel every detail, even the serrated edges and frayed tips that some of them had. It was amazing! I looked over the expanse of the field and thought, I am everything. This is all me – this is all a construct of my own mind!

Then I saw a low-lying grey brick wall near the hedge and I ran my hands across it. I could feel every indent in the cement between the bricks and every imperfection in the grain of the stone. The detail was astonishing!

'This is all me! I am one with everything! It's all a dream!' I said to myself.

While I had been doing all this, the coachload of shadow aspects (which I had kind of forgotten about) had pulled up and now I found myself being attacked by three of them. As they attacked me, I embraced them firmly, all three of them in one big bear hug, as I yelled, 'I am one with you! We are all one!'

Once they heard this, it seemed that they had been fully embraced and they actually became quite friendly. I wanted them to appreciate the empty nature of the dream, too, so I said to them, 'Hey, guys, look at this.' I began to tap my fingers on the hard surface of the wall, saying, 'This wall looks and feels totally solid, right? But

249

because I know that I'm dreaming, I can push my hand into it. This wall is emptiness.'

My hand passed easily through it. The befriended shadow aspects watched on eagerly.

Then I woke myself up.

Prep before Bed

Twenty minutes of meditation on reversed red Tibetan 'ah' before bed. Prayers to HH Karmapa to get lucid.

Dream 8: Teachings from Lama Yeshe Rinpoche
31 December 2007

I dreamed that I had just fallen off a cliff and the sense of falling became a lucidity trigger, and I realized that I was dreaming. I managed to hover in mid-air before I hit the ground. With full lucidity, I flew into a modern-looking Moroccan-style living room, thought, I must get teachings from Lama Yeshe, and willed him to appear.

Instantly a human form appeared on the sofa in front of me. It looked plain-faced, like a blank canvas of human form. I prayed for Lama Yeshe to enter this form and soon he started to appear within it. Eventually the entire form transformed into Lama Yeshe. There he was, sitting on the sofa in front of me, clear as day.

I said to him, 'Lama Yeshe, what meditation practices should I do?'

He confidently replied, 'Given that you have one and a half hours [a day?], 45 minutes for dream practice and 45 minutes for waking practice, you should do 45 minutes waking practice many times and then you will gain control over the six channels.'

As he spoke, he looked into a golden bowl full of dark liquid that was on a coffee table in front of him, and golden images were formed on the surface of the liquid, illustrating what he was telling me. I saw an Eye of Buddha symbol and an African mask being traced in gold on the surface of the liquid.

Still fully lucid, I continued to receive teachings from Lama Yeshe, but when I asked him to explain more, he vanished into thin air like a ghost in a movie.

I woke myself up and wrote this all down. Was it really him or just a projection of my own inner guru archetype? Not sure, but in the waking state the teachings still seem valid, so I guess that's all that matters.

Dream 9: Shadow Integration Lucid Dream
10 March 2009

I dreamed that I was walking along a street with a friend. I turned to him and said, 'This feels so much like a dream, doesn't it? I'd better check, just in case it actually is.'

I then proceeded to do a hand reality check, my hand changed and I became lucid. I was so surprised that I felt I needed to do an extra check just to be sure, so I looked at my hand and willed it to get smaller, which it did. I then willed it to get bigger, which it did.

Then I walked off the street and into a nearby room, which had about four or five different people in it. One of them looked quite scary. Knowing that all of these people were personifications of my psyche, I went around the room hugging each one of them as per usual. When I got to the scary-looking one (a big fat man dressed in a kind of police uniform), he seemed very aggressive and it dawned on me that he was a full-on shadow aspect. As I went to hug him, he bit me hard on my neck and whispered hateful stuff in my ear. His bite really hurt me and I had a flash of anger before I regained my composure and realized that this was all a dream and that he was my shadow, the representation of my repressed capacity for violence and wrath, and so to try to fight him with anger was pure folly.

Then the shadow aspect spoke again, saying, 'You will never be able to stop me biting – I am the essence of violence! Violence is my nature!'

I was so scared, but I realized that I had to embrace him. I couldn't hug him, so I would have to try something new. I grabbed him and wrestled him to the floor. Then I kneeled over him and began literally to inhale him, to breathe in the essence of this darkness, to integrate this energy that I had repressed. I breathed in all the denied anger and disowned power that he contained.

As I did this, he began to dissolve in front of my very eyes. It was still quite scary because I could actually feel the dark energy that he embodied entering me, but I knew that the shadow couldn't hurt me if my motivation was to integrate it.

As I continued to breathe in the shadow's essence, I repeated out loud, 'I am integrated, I am balanced, I am joy, love and equanimity. I am integrated, I am balanced, I am joy, love and equanimity,' and the shadow continued to shrink and dissolve into the vapour that I was inhaling.

Once the shadow had totally dissolved, I stood up and said, in a low, wrathful voice, 'That was a good thing. Now I can be fully integrated.'

Then I woke up.

Prep before Bed

Fell asleep at about midnight doing the 'I. Am I dreaming? 2. Am I dreaming?' FAC technique. Also briefly prayed to Guru Rinpoche for a lucid dream.

Dream 10: Lucid Meditation
24 July 2003

I got lucid and began to fly around the dreamscape. I remembered my current dream plan: to try to meditate in a lucid dream!

I flew up to the top of a very tall pillar and got into meditation posture. I was so excited. I'd wanted to try meditating in a lucid dream for ages, but always seemed to get involved in something else (sex usually!) before I could.

As I sat on top of the pillar, I started to watch my breath and meditate. Within seconds, my mind began to blow. I entered into an experience of bliss (or what I think bliss is like!) followed by an intense rushing feeling. I thought my brain was going to explode; it was like normal meditation x 1,000!

Then I heard the voice of my friend Carlos, like a sports commentator, say, 'The meditation is becoming too powerful to comprehend,' which worried me a bit, so I managed to bring myself back to my dream body and out of the meditation.

I then flew down from the pillar into a town that seemed to be somewhere in Tibet or Nepal. When the people in the town looked at me, they either stared in shock or they covered their eyes. Their reaction scared me a bit, so I woke up.

I lay in bed buzzing. That was so cool! I hadn't prepared myself for something as intense as that. Next time I'm gonna recite mantras and see if I can invoke buddhas.

Dream 11: Galantamine Lucidity!
2 November 2011

Woke at 5 a.m. and did short blessing ritual and prayers for protection during my Galantamine experience. I then took two 4mg caps of Galantamine and did ten minutes of meditation at my shrine.

Got into bed and spent about 15 mins just watching the hypnagogic and then literally watched the Galantamine set in. So weird! Did FAC and ended up in false awakening. I became fully lucid and started to assess the situation.

Although my bedroom looked very realistic, the lucidity was actually quite cloudy. I thought to myself, I'll do some meditation! So I turned to my shrine, which was just by my bed, as it is in reality. But although everything in the room looked identical to waking reality, one thing had changed: my shrine had been ransacked! It had been smashed up and there was weird childish graffiti scrawled across the faces of the Buddha paintings.

Even within the lucid dream I knew instantly what this meant: Galantamine vandalizes the spiritual aspect of your unconscious. Everything in the dream was a representation of me, and my inner shrine had been ransacked.

I woke up.

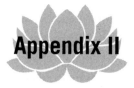

Appendix II

A Selection of Lucid Dreams, Clarity Dreams and Hypnopompic Insights

In this final appendix, I'm presenting a collection of some of the most interesting lucid dreams, clarity dreams and hypnopompic insights that I've experienced over the past ten years or so. There's even the odd OBE thrown in there, too.

Although, as Rob Nairn always says, 'There's nothing more boring than hearing about other people's dreams,' hopefully these lucid dreams won't bore you too much, as I've tried to include only the juiciest ones!

Dream 12: Buddha Nature Lucid!
11th January 2010

I dreamed that I threw a dog's paw through a first-storey apartment window, an act so bizarre that I habitually did a reality check: I tried to read some text on a sign in the courtyard of the apartment block, but it was all jumbled and so I knew I was dreaming.

Now fully lucid, I flew up into the overcast evening sky and engaged my current dream plan by calling out to the sky, 'I want to meet my Buddha nature. Show me my Buddha nature!'

Then I looked down at the ground, expecting to see a monk or wise man or some other archetypal representation of my Buddha nature. Nobody appeared, but suddenly the cloudy evening sky became illuminated by a bright orange glow, as if the sun had just risen to its highest point.

'What about my Buddha nature? I want to meet my Buddha nature!' I complained, until it clicked: I was meeting my Buddha nature! This was it! My Buddha nature was illumination, bright light in an evening sky, sunlight from behind the clouds, a luminous glow!

I was then joined by two or three other people, and we flew over the desert terrain towards the sun before I woke up feeling totally blissed out.

Prep before Bed

Fell asleep after 6 a.m. Wake-up reciting the script of the dream plan: 'In my next lucid dream I meet my Buddha nature.' I had also been to teachings on Buddha nature that evening and was sleeping in the spare room at Mum's house (different bed = good for lucidity).

Dream 13: Lecture Composed in Lucid Dream

19 July 2011

Before bed I had been thinking about what I wanted to talk about at my upcoming 'Secret Garden Party' slot. I had thought that the concept of Oneness and how it related to lucid dreaming seemed like a good subject, but it was too late to work on it, so I went to bed.

I then spent the entire night dreaming about the concept of Oneness and actually ended up writing a talk about it within a lucid dream! I had five different dreams in fact, but all were about writing and performing a new talk on Oneness. I wrote almost the entire talk in the dreams, rehearsed it and even showed it to dream characters who gave me feedback and advice. The first dream, which was lucid/witnessing, even gave me an original title: 'Oneness: from

Theory to Practice', and told me that it should be about ten minutes long and must start with the line 'I wrote this talk in a dream' and finish with the question 'If everything is Oneness, why bother?' (How very nihilistic!)

Dream 14: Shadow Integration
8 January 2008

This was the first time that I ever consciously integrated my shadow within a lucid dream and it's the dream that I referenced in my 2011 TED talk. It represented a turning point in my dream practice and the start of a colourful relationship with my shadow that continues today.

After a false awakening I dreamed that I was being cornered in a dark outside car park by three menacing figures, two men and one woman. They were radiating malicious intent and the fear made me become lucid. I called out, 'Dream! This is all a dream!', to which they answered, 'So what? You're still dreaming!'

I was getting scared now, so I yelled, 'It's a dream, so I can control it! Stop, stop!' But they didn't stop, they just seemed to coalesce into one big three-headed demon.

They said, 'You can't control this!' and closed in on me, laughing at my fear.

Then, just before I was going to attack them in self-defence, I remembered what Rob Nairn had told me about dealing with the shadow. He had said that instead of fighting it in my dreams, I should embrace it and talk to it.

I called out loud, 'Shadow, my shadow!' and then wrapped my arms round the three-headed demon.

I could feel it struggling within my embrace and then a heavy metal soundtrack suddenly started playing, with the repeated vocal refrain: 'This is how you become five again. This is how you become shadow, shadow.'

As the music played, I dissolved into a green triangle of light and then the entire dreamscape, including the shadow aspects, dissolved too. It felt as though I was regressing back into the past, or back into the void, where I would meet the source of my shadow.

The next thing I knew, the three-headed shadow aspect had transformed, through my embrace, into me. I was standing in front of a direct carbon copy of myself – facing my own true self. This was the source of my shadow – not a demon, but me, of course.

Prep before Bed

Had just read Rob Nairn's letter asking me to teach lucid dreaming sometime in the future – very exciting! Had jet-lag due to a flight back from India = REM rebound. Had also watched *Dawn of the Dead* before bed = nightmares.

Dream 15: Sleeping Body OBE in Locale 1
10 November 2012

I was teaching in Jersey and after being in a hyper-alert mental and vibrational state, I finally got to sleep – or so I thought.

After feeling far too energized to sleep, eventually I seemed to be entering some sort of lucid dream, but then I felt a vibrational energy that swept up my legs, especially around my calves, and I knew that I was about to have an OBE. I found myself whisked off into the blackness. The next thing I knew I was a disembodied point of awareness looking at my body on the bed. A Locale 1 OBE! I had been trying to do this for months and I thought to myself, This is it. I'm looking at my sleeping body in an OBE!

Then I got a bit freaked out and suddenly I found myself in my own bedroom in London looking down at Jade sleeping. As she slept, I used my intent to try to move the covers off her as a form of communication from the OBE state. When I tried this, she seemed to become disturbed, so I used my energy form to try to smooth her hair to reassure her and yet still hopefully to signal that it was me in OBE form. Then I said her name and asked if she could see me. I told her that I was in the room in Jersey, but she didn't reply. It seemed that my energy form could disturb her if it touched her body on the bed but my voice could not be heard.

I woke up/returned to my body at about 1:45 a.m. after getting to bed at 12:45 a.m.

Prep before Bed

Two and a half hours of meditation today, plus energy-body shifting exercises and sleeping in an unfamiliar bed.

Dream 16: One Hundred-Syllable Mantra Lucid Dream
23 December 2010

This was one of the most memorable lucid dreams I have ever had. It went on for so long, contained so many different elements – everything from mantra recitation to shadow integration – and had such a funny musical-theatre ending that it still makes me laugh!

I dreamed that I was discussing with a nun how crazy it was that I might be in a dream and that at one point I might wake up in a bed in a future world and find that everything had been a dream. Then I realized that I was actually dreaming right then!

I looked around and saw that I was in a huge empty hall, as big as a warehouse. I did hand reality checks, got fully lucid and engaged my current dream plan of chanting the 100-syllable purification mantra within the lucid dream.

As I began to chant, I could feel a huge movement of energy and soon I saw loads of people rushing towards me from each end of the huge space. Suddenly I felt a flash of fear and thought, Oh God, I'm chanting a purification mantra so I'm going to invoke loads of shadow aspects! But then, as they came closer, I saw that they were in fact all maroon-robed monks and nuns. There were hundreds of them, all flocking into the hall, beckoned by the mantra. Within a few seconds, they had assembled and sat down in rows, and a chant master had appeared on a fully kitted-out stage with musicians playing the tune of the chant and they were all chanting along with me in unison! All these projections of my own mind chanting together!

I saw that Lama Yeshe Rinpoche had appeared, too, and was sitting on a high throne facing the stage. Still totally lucid, I went over to him and asked if I could sit in the empty space next to him. He seemed to be in deep meditation, but nodded in affirmation. So there I sat, on the right-hand side of Lama Yeshe, with hundreds of Tibetan monks and nuns all chanting the 100-syllable mantra together within the lucid dream! Amazing!

Soon after this, I heard more people arriving, not monks and nuns, but projections of everyday people, and some of my shadow aspects (sexualized/angry-looking people), who had heard the call of the purification mantra, too, but, unlike the monks and nuns, weren't there to sit quietly! The shadow aspects were there for trouble!

I turned round and started to chant at the shadow aspects directly, which seemed to rile them even more. They didn't like my attempt to purify them! So I waded into the crowd of shadow aspects and started hugging them and integrating them through hugs and telling them that I loved them. I just kept going up to the most offensive-looking ones and kissing them with love.

Then I became super-lucid as I remembered that in lucid dreams we are one with everything, even with inanimate objects. I had knocked over a chair during a fracas with a shadow aspect, so I went and picked it up and actually started hugging and kissing it! I was ecstatic in the knowledge that I was inside my own head and that the more love and appreciation that I could show to each and every thing, the more loving and appreciative my mind would become in waking life!

Throughout all this, the monks and nuns had continued to chant the 100-syllable mantra and so I decided to make my way up to the stage where the chant master and musicians were leading the chant. When I got up on stage, they stopped the music and chanting and I found myself facing the audience of about 500 monks and nuns and a few hundred everyday dream characters and shadow aspects. I saw a dream character who I knew was a representation of a deeply beneficial part of my unconscious and I wanted him to get up on stage so that I could thank him. As I took the mic, the band started up as if they wanted me to sing, and the crowd was calling for a song, too!

Still lucid and totally aware that this was all a dream, I started to sing from my heart, 'I love you all! I really do! I love you all! I love you so much!' I sang it over and over, and soon the whole room was singing it together! All these aspects of my own psyche were singing, 'I love you so I love you so much!' to a tune of 'da dee da dee, da dee dee da dee'! It was so funny, but so beautiful too that my unconscious mind became an expression of pure love! I was crying and calling out over the singing, 'Make me kinder! Make my more loving! Make me more beneficial! I love you all! Thank you so much!'

I woke up crying with joy, totally blissful.

Prep before Bed

Kickboxing energy drink led to restless sleep, read Théun Mares' Toltec book before bed, went to bed on an empty stomach, lunar eclipse last night. Sleeping on sofa at Mum's place. Been doing a lot more Vajrasattva purification practice in the past two weeks.

Dream 17: Lucid Self-Manifestation as Chenrezig
28 February 2007

I became spontaneously lucid and remembered the instructions that Lama Yeshe had given me two weeks before about taking on the form of Chenrezig Buddha in a lucid dream. So, with full lucidity, I said the mantra of Chenrezig, Om mani peme hung, and then looked down expectantly to see if I had taken on the form of Chenrezig, but I hadn't.

The lucidity was crystal-clear, though. I was flying high up above the world, reciting the Om mani peme hung mantra and consciously dedicating it to the wellbeing of all the people below and it felt very powerful.

I then landed back on the ground and worked through the visualization of the four-armed form of Chenrezig point by point. Strangely, I could remember exactly where each arm was positioned and what each arm held – something I'm rubbish at in waking life! Although I couldn't see it because my eyes were closed during the visualization, I could feel that I was physically taking on the form of Chenrezig. Again I flew up into the sky and recited the Mani mantra for the benefit of all beings, but this time I was in the actual form of the four-armed Chenrezig.

Suddenly I felt the presence of doom or pure darkness mocking me and challenging me. I was still flying and reciting the Om mani peme hung mantra, but this time incredibly quickly, far more quickly than I could ever recite it in real life. Quicker and quicker and quicker it went, until the intensity started to make the lucidity slip and the dreamscape completely transformed.

I was now in a totally new dreamscape in the body of a small child walking in a procession of adults, still 100 per cent lucid. One of the adults in the procession in front of me turned around and smiled at me. As he turned, I saw that it was Lama Yeshe!

Dream 18: Teachings on Pain and Suffering
12th November 2010

I became lucid gradually in a dream in which I was on the New Year's Eve retreat with Tim Freke (a gnostic scholar). He said, 'You now know that you are dreaming and I will guide you through the lucid dream.' This comment brought me to full lucidity, as I realized that I was actually already lucid and this was all a dream!

Then, without warning, Tim produced a huge flaming log of wood and smashed it over my back as I stood next to him in front of the group. The burning embers shattered and poured down my back and onto the floor around my feet. I felt the intense pain of the burning coals as they singed my skin and scorched my back. I realized that this must be some sort of upright 'fire-walking' demonstration. Tim said it was 'a teaching about the difference between pain and suffering'.

The pain felt so real, but as the group stood around me, watching the burning embers scorch my skin, Tim looked at me with a kind face and smiled. With that smile, I realized what this demonstration was about. I felt pain because I had had a burning log smashed over my back, but I felt no suffering because I knew that this was all a dream. I was fully aware that the pain was merely a projection of my own mind and that suffering was caused by aversion to pain, not by pain itself.

In the lucid dream I could feel pain and yet I wasn't suffering – this is what Tim was teaching me. He was explaining this to the group as I stood there and they all seemed to understand it.

I also realized that pain in the waking state was illusory and that so much of our suffering was often self-inflicted, due to our powerful rejection of all pain and discomfort.

Once the demonstration was over, Tim asked me to help 'polish and clean everybody's light bulbs' and we proceeded to go down the line of people polishing their light bulbs, which seemed somehow to be an outward expression of their consciousness.

Prep before Bed

Woke at 11:58 p.m. after going to bed at 10:10 p.m. and falling asleep reciting, 'I want to recognize my dreams and realize the awareness that lies beyond my projections.' I also spent a few hours before bed reading Tim's book (*The Laughing Jesus* by Timothy Freke and Peter Gandy).

Dream 19: Guru Rinpoche Self-manifestation and Lama Yeshe OBE!

21 November 2011

Lucid dream after 4:30 a.m. Wake-up. Using FAC method, I went straight into a dream and looked at my hands once lucid. I then engaged my dream plan of calling out the long invocation mantra of Guru Rinpoche. I called it out three times so loudly I thought I might have even been calling out in my sleep, and then I began levitating into the air and transforming into Guru Rinpoche.

It was a slow transformation into the form of Guru Rinpoche, but I actually manifested his ornaments and everything. It felt very powerful and very stable.

After this, I floated up and saw a computer screen with an outer-space screensaver on it, so I used it as a portal by climbing into it and thus into the space scene that it depicted.

Once in space, I engaged the OBE practice and called out, 'Out of body now! Lama Yeshe Rinpoche now!' and got whizzed off at great speed into the pitch-black space. I was going very fast through several layers/slices of space and it seemed as though I was passing through the very fabric of the universe.

Then suddenly I arrived in a kind of office space with little cubicles and desks, but quite big, open-plan, very solid, very OBE, not lucid-dreamlike at all.

As soon as I arrived, a big, fat African guy ran up to me and hugged me. He seemed very surprised to see me, but happy nonetheless. I then realized that it was Lama Yeshe Rinpoche!

After the initial greeting he seemed to think that I had come at a not-so-perfect time and he politely made his excuses. It seemed that I had arrived unannounced and that although he was happy to see me, it was not a good time for him. Maybe it was because he was in the form of a fat African guy? God, OBEs are so weird!

Prep before Bed

Ngondro practice dedicated to 'Give me a lucid dream so powerful that it changes everything, for the benefit of all beings!' And lots of prayers and true confidence that I would get lucid. Woke at 4:30 a.m. then did FAC perfectly and prayers, including long invocation mantra as I fell asleep with a visualization of Guru Rinpoche and Lama Yeshe in my heart centre.

Dream 20: Lama Yeshe Clarity Dream
19 January 2010

I was at some sort of boatyard and had broken my leg and was losing a lot of blood. Even so, I felt fearless and was determined not to die and to get myself to safety. I was dragging myself along wooden decking to the edge of the boatyard, where there was a ferry waiting to take me to the other side of the harbour and to safety.

Then suddenly I saw Lama Yeshe Rinpoche over by the ferry crossing, just standing there waiting happily. I didn't want to cause a fuss or disturb him, so I simply greeted him warmly as I hauled myself still bleeding onto the ferry boat.

Once I was aboard, Lama Yeshe asked me, 'Where are you going?'

I replied, 'I've broken my leg, Lama, and I need to get to the other side or I might die.'

He cheerfully acknowledged my situation by saying, 'Oh I see! Yes, OK then,' as I floated off on the ferry boat. Then he smiled broadly and called out to me, 'Don't worry, I will bring you over. It will happen subtly at first and there won't be lots of chances, but I will bring you over.'

Dream 21: Amazing Clarity Dream with Dilgo Khyentse Rinpoche

May 2003

I never met Dilgo Khyentse Rinpoche – he died in 1991 – and although I knew that this dream was special, it has taken years of dream yoga practice for me to truly appreciate just how important it was for me. Whether it was just an egotistical projection from my 19-year-old mind or whether it really was my inner guru who spoke to me, I still don't know, and perhaps it doesn't really matter because this dream has served as a source of beneficial inspiration for me ever since.

After the Sogyal Rinpoche Easter retreat I prayed before bed to meet Dilgo Khyentse Rinpoche in my next dream and that's exactly what happened.

In the dream there was a big fight as well as some sort of sexual aspect and then Dilgo Khyentse Rinpoche appeared.

He looked at me with a sort of loving disapproval, like a loving mother who's caught a child being naughty, as if he was a bit disappointed at having been invoked in such a violent dream, but he was still quite happy looking. I tried to reassure him by saying, 'You are a great master and I won't confuse the man with the lama,' and then he smiled and replied, 'For only two lifetimes I have been calling you, but now you have heard. You have good potential.'

I woke up crying.

A SELECTION OF HYPNOPOMPIC INSIGHTS

Hypnopompic insights are flashes of insight that occur just as we come out of sleep and dreams but before we fully wake up, open our eyes and engage the waking state. Sometimes they present themselves as punchlines to the dream we were just having, other times they are more like pithy commentaries on the dream and often they are seemingly unrelated flashes of insight which arrive fully formed from a seemingly unknown place. I believe that they are available to us all if we can just wake up with a bit more awareness and listen to the echo of our dreams. Here are a few of my favourites from recent years:

21 January 2009
After going to bed worrying about the clothes I had worn to teach in, I woke in the morning with a flash of insight that said: 'Mud on your shoes means that you have communed with nature. This is a sacred communion that you should never be ashamed of.'

10 January 2010
As my alarm clock sounded, a seemingly disembodied voice said, 'Take this and use it to wipe your eyes when you feel the sadness that only a traveller knows: to have no roots, to have no home.'

19 November 2011
At the end of the dream I saw a sign that said: 'If you don't salivate when you think about your job or your wife, get a new job and get a new wife.'

9 January 2009
The first thought that I had in the morning came fully formed: 'We are so concerned with what happened back then or what's gonna happen when, but what about the now? Let's do now.'

22 December 2011
Just as I was waking I heard the punchline of the dream. It was: 'It's all about widening your bandwidth. Meditation broadens your bandwidth so your download speed is more efficient and your computer works more smoothly.'

30 August 2010

In the tiny moment between waking up and getting out of bed the following insight dawned on me, voiced by a ·seemingly disembodied voice which was not my own: 'We are limited by everyday things but if we could only learn to see beyond them there is great benefit to be gained.'

6 August 2011

After an intense lucid dream, the flash of an idea came to me as I woke up: 'For every death you experience, you gain an extra lane on your highway.'

1 May 2011

As the dream faded from my mind's eye and the sunlight streamed through my eyelids, I heard a voice say: 'To keep doing what you've always done, to stick to the path, to keep to what you know, that's not going to change much. But to do something new, to take a new path, that's really how you change something.'

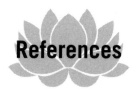

References

Chapter 1: The Basics

1. Frederik van Eeden, 'A study of dreams', *Proceedings of the Society for Psychical Research* 26, 1913, 431–61

2. Cited in Michael Katz, *Tibetan Dream Yoga*, Bodhi Tree, 2011, p.3

3. U. Voss, R. Holzmann, I. Tuin, J. A. Hobson, 'Lucid dreaming: a state of consciousness with features of both waking and non-lucid dreaming', *Sleep* 32 (9), September 2009, 1191–200

4. Max-Planck-Gesellschaft, 'Lucid dreamers help scientists locate the seat of meta-consciousness in the brain', ScienceDaily, 27 July 2012. Retrieved 10 August 2012 from http://www.sciencedaily.com/releases/2012/07/120727095555.htm

5. Albert Einstein, Letter to Robert S. Marcus, 12 February 1950, The Albert Einstein Archives, Hebrew University of Jerusalem

6. Robert Waggoner, *Lucid Dreaming*, Moment Point Press, 2009, p.17

7. Ibid., p.20

8. Rob Preece, *The Psychology of Buddhist Tantra*, Snow Lion Publications, 2012, p.107

9. J. Allan Hobson, *Dreaming*, Oxford University Press, 2005, p.126

10. Francisco J. Varela and HH Dalai Lama, *Sleeping, Dreaming, and Dying*, Wisdom Publications, 1997, p.105

11. Ibid., p.106

Chapter 2: Where Science and Spirituality Meet

1.	Keith Hearne, *The Dream Machine*, The Aquarian Press, 1990, p.12
2.	Paul and Charla Devereux, *Lucid Dreaming*, Daily Grail Publishing, 2011, p.76
3.	LaBerge, S., Nagel, L., Dement, W. & Zarcone, V. (1981a). 'Lucid dreaming verified by volitional communication during REM sleep'. *Perceptual and Motor Skills*, 52, 727–732.
4.	Stephen Batchelor, 'Buddhism for this One and Only Life', the first talk of his *Tricycle* online retreat, 26 June 2010
5.	Trinlay Tulku Rinpoche, 'East is West', *Tricycle* magazine online, Summer 2005, p.5
6.	The *Pali Vinaya*, Oldenberg, I.295, quoted in Serenity Young, *Dreaming in the Lotus*, Wisdom Publications, 1999, p.44
7.	Francisco J. Varela and HH Dalai Lama, *Sleeping, Dreaming, and Dying*, Wisdom Publications, 1997, p.45

Chapter 3: Why Do We Dream?

1.	J. Allan Hobson, *Dreaming*, Oxford University Press, 2005, p.52
2.	Fraser Boa, *The Way of the Dream*, Windrose, 1988, p.16
3.	Rob Nairn, *Living, Dreaming, Dying*, Shambhala Publications, 2004, p.41
4.	C. G. Jung, *Dreams*, trans. R. F. C. Hull, Princeton University Press, 1974, p.3
5.	Nairn, op. cit.
6.	Ibid.
7.	B. Alan Wallace, *Dreaming Yourself Awake*, Shambhala, 2012, p. 68
8.	Francisco J. Varela and HH Dalai Lama, *Sleeping, Dreaming, and Dying*, Wisdom Publications, 1997, p.42

Chapter 4: The Benefits of Lucid Dreaming and Mindfulness of Dream & Sleep

1.	Valerie Austin, *Self-Hypnosis*, Thorsons, 1994, p.26
2.	Ibid., p.27
3.	Marc Barasch, *Healing Dreams*, Riverhead, 2000

4. www.cancer.org/Treatment/TreatmentsandSideEffects/
   ComplementaryandAlternativeMedicine/MindBodyandSpirit/
   imagery

5. Michael Katz, *Tibetan Dream Yoga*, Bodhi Tree, 2011, p.31

6. www.dw-world.de/dw/article/0,,2040400,00.html

7. Luke Behncke, 'Mental skills training for sports: a brief review',
   Athletic Insight: The Online Journal of Sport Psychology 6(1), March
   2004

8. http://sportsmedicine.about.com/od/sportspsychology/a/
   thinkstrong.htm

9. www.telegraph.co.uk/news/worldnews/northamerica/
   usa/1363146/Thinking-about-exercise-can-beef-up-biceps.html

10. Katz, op. cit., p.37

11. Silvio Scarone from the Università degli Studi di Milano, speaking
    at a European Science Foundation meeting in 2009: www.esf.
    org/activities/exploratory-workshops/news/ext-news-singleview/
    article/new-links-between-dreams-and-psychosis-could-revive-
    dream-therapy-in-psychiatry-585.html

12. C. G. Jung, 'Psychology and Religion', 1938, in Collected Works 11:
    Psychology and Religion: West and East, Princeton University Press,
    1975, p.131

13. W. B. Yeats, *Responsibilities*, Cuala Press, 1914, p.172, attributed to
    an 'old play'

14. Dzogchen Ponlop Rinpoche, *Mind Beyond Death*, Snow Lion
    Publications, 2008, p.1

15. Katz, op. cit., p.103

16. B. Alan Wallace, *Dreaming Yourself Awake*, Shambhala Publications,
    2012, p.20

17. Chokyi Nyingma Rinpoche, Rigpa, London, 2010

18. Dzigar Kongtrul Rinpoche, *It's Up to You*, Shambhala Publications,
    2006, p.12

19. Wallace, op. cit., p.77

20. Rob Nairn in conversation with the author, August 2011.

21. Marcus Chown, cosmology consultant of the *New Scientist*: http://
    www.telegraph.co.uk/science/6546462/The-10-weirdest-physics-
    facts-from-relativity-to-quantum physics.html

22. Cited in Michael Katz, *Tibetan Dream Yoga*, Bodhi Tree, 2011, p.120
23. Bhante Henepola Gunaratana, 'Mindfulness and concentration', *Tricycle* online magazine, Fall 1998
24. Rob Nairn, teaching at Kagyu Samye Dzong Buddhist Centre, London, 2009
25. Dr Akong Rinpoche, interview with the author, 2009
26. Timothy Freke, teaching at Glastonbury Abbey, December 2010
27. http://www.tricycle.com/daily-dharma/wake-world
28. Tenzin Wangyal Rinpoche, video teaching: http://www.youtube.com/watch?v=6Gls65GDMGQ
29. http://news.harvard.edu/gazette/story/2010/11/wandering-mind-not-a-happy-mind/
30. Freke, op. cit.

Chapter 5: Lucid Dreaming Techniques

1. Dzogchen Ponlop Rinpoche, *Mind Beyond Death*, Snow Lion Publications, 2008, footnote 10
2. http://www.psychoanalysis.org.uk/solms4.htm
3. Lama Surya Das, *Tibetan Dream Yoga*, audio CD, Sounds True, 2001
4. Richard Wiseman, *59 Seconds*, Pan, 2010, p.16
5. Carlos Castaneda, *Journey to Ixtlan*, Simon and Schuster, 1972, p.114
6. Ibid.
7. http://www.lucidity.com/LucidDreamingFAQ2.html
8. Jill Bolte Taylor, *My Stroke of Insight*, Hodder and Stoughton, 2008
9. http://www.lucidity.com/NL53.ResearchPastFuture.html
10. Daniel Love, *Are You Dreaming?*, Enchanted Loom Publishing, 2013, p.2
11. Ibid.
12. Ibid., p.83
13. Michael Katz, *Tibetan Dream Yoga*, Bodhi Tree, 2011, p.67, commenting on Gyaltrul Rinpoche, *Ancient Wisdom*, Snow Lion Publications, 1993, p.80
14. http://www.lucidity.com/LucidDreamingFAQ2.html
15. www.lucidity.com/NL63.RU.Naps.html

16. B. Alan Wallace, *Dreaming Yourself Awake*, Shambhala Publications, 2012, p.30

17. Tibetan Buddhist nun and author Bhikshuni Thubten Chodron, http://www.tricycle.com/feature/meditators-toolbox

Chapter 6: Mindfulness of Dream & Sleep Techniques

1. B. Alan Wallace, *Dreaming Yourself Awake*, Shambhala Publications, 2012, p.102

2. Akong Tulku Rinpoche in conversation with the author.

3. [Studies' refs t/c in] Richard Wiseman, *59 Seconds*, Pan, 2010

4. Tenzin Wangyal Rinpoche, video teaching from www.ligmincha. org/retreats/dream-yoga.html

5. Dzogchen Ponlop Rinpoche, *Mind Beyond Death*, Snow Lion Publications, 2008

6. Patrul Rinpoche, *Words of My Perfect Teacher*, Shambhala, 1994, pp.403, 410

7. Rob Nairn, *Living, Dreaming, Dying*, Shambhala Publications, 2004, p.38

8. Timothy Freke, 'Lucid Living' teachings, December 2009

9. Francisco J. Varela, with HH Dalai Lama, *Sleeping, Dreaming, and Dying*, Wisdom Publications, 1997, p.40

10. Traleg Kyabgon Rinpoche, Dream Yoga, five-disc DVD, E-Vam Buddhist Institute, 2008

11. Cited in B. Alan Wallace, *Dreaming Yourself Awake*, Shambhala Publications, 2012, p.99

12. http://internationalreporter.com/News-1803/study-ties-drop-in-deaths-to-a-little-nap-after-lunch.html

13. www.healingtao.org/deutsch/artikel2.htm

14. www.ncbi.nlm.nih.gov/pubmed/16540232

15. www.timesonline.co.uk/tol/life_and_style/health/expert_advice/article3817673.ece

16. Karl Doghramji, MD, 'Melatonin and its receptors: a new class of sleep-promoting agents', http://ukpmc.ac.uk/articlerender. cgi?artid=1257932

Chapter 7: Going Deeper into Mindfulness of Dream & Sleep

1. Carlos Castaneda, *Journey to Ixtlan*, Simon and Schuster, 1972, p.198
2. Mingyur Rinpoche, public talk, London, 2005
3. Jeff Warren, *Head Trip*, Oneworld Publications, 2009, p. 39
4. Richard Wiseman, *59 Seconds*, Pan, 2010, p.119
5. Cited in Deirdre Barrett's *The Committee of Sleep*, Crown, 2001
6. In conversation with the author, 2012.
7. Krishnamurti, *The Beginnings of Learning*, Krishnamurti Foundation Trust, 1979
8. www.tricycle.com/online-retreats/green-meditation/recovery-dark
9. www.menshealth.com/yoga/livingwell/How_to_Sleep_Right_Tonight.php+wake+up+every+90+minutes
10. Namgyal Rinpoche, *The Womb of Form*, Bodhi Publishing, 1998, p.73
11. http://www.drweil.com/drw/u/ART00521/three-breathing-exercises.html
12. Ibid.
13. Traleg Kyabgon Rinpoche, *Dream Yoga,* five-disc DVD set, E-Vam Buddhist Institute, 2008
14. Michael Katz, *Tibetan Dream Yoga*, Bodhi Tree, 2011, p.28.
15. Traleg Kyabgon Rinpoche, op. cit.
16. N. Krause, 'Praying for Others, Financial Strain and Physical Health Status in Later Life' (2003), cited in Richard Wiseman, *59 Seconds*, Pan, 2010, p.188.
17. Glenn H. Mullin, *Six Yogas of Naropa: Tsongkhapa's Commentary entitled: A Book of Three Inspirations*, Snow Lion Publications, 2005.
18. Cited in B. Alan Wallace, *Dreaming Yourself Awake*, Shambhala, 2012, p.99
19. Lama Surya Das, *Tibetan Dream Yoga*, audio CD, Sounds True, 2001
20. Carlos Castaneda, *Journey to Ixtlan*, Simon and Schuster, 1972, p.127
21. www.tibetanmedicine-edu.org/pdf/dreamsD1.pdf
22. http://dreamstudies.org/2009/09/02/what-is-lucid-dreaming/

23. www.telegraph.co.uk/health/healthnews/5070874/Reading-can-help-reduce-stress.html

24. Tenzin Wangyal Rinpoche, public talk, London, November 2012

25. Lama Zangmo in conversation with the author, May 2011

Chapter 8: 'I'm Lucid – What Now?'

1. B. Alan Wallace, *Dreaming Yourself Awake*, Shambhala Publications, 2012, p.102

2. Robert Waggoner, *Lucid Dreaming*, Moment Point Press, 2009, p.31

3. In conversation with the author.

4. Jill Bolte Taylor, PhD, *My Stroke of Insight*, Hodder and Stoughton, 2008, p.30

5. Valerie Austin, *Self-Hypnosis*, Thorsons, 1994, p.69

6. Rob Nairn, in conversation with the author, 2010.

7. http://www.bbc.co.uk/iplayer/episode/b00xxgbn/Horizon_20102011_What_Is_Reality/

8. Akong Tulku Rinpoche, in conversation with the author, 2009.

9. Namkhai Norbu Rinpoche, *The Cycle of Day and Night*, Barrytown/Stationhill Press, 1987

10. http://www.ted.com/talks/ben_goldacre_battling_bad_science.html

11. B. Alan Wallace, teaching at the Kagyu Samye Dzong Buddhist centre, London, June 2012

12. Glenn H. Mullin, *Six Yogas of Naropa: Tsongkhapa's Commentary entitled: A Book of Three Inspirations*, Snow Lion Publications, 2005.

13. Akong Tulku Rinpoche, in conversation with the author, 2009.

14. C. G. Jung, *The Archetypes and the Collective Unconscious* (The Collected Works of C.G. Jung, Vol.9, Part 1)., Routledge and Kegan Paul, 1959

15. Geshe Lhundrup Sopa, *Peacocks in the Poison Grove*, Wisdom Publications, 1996

16. C.G. Jung, 'The Importance of the Unconscious in Psychopathology', *The British Medical Journal*, vol. 2, no. 2,814 (5 December 1914), 964–8

17. William Shakespeare, *The Tempest*, Act V, scene i, 267–76

18. Deepak Chopra, *The Shadow*, DVD, Hay House, 2009

19. Lama Surya Das, *Tibetan Dream Yoga*, audio CD, Sounds True, 2001

20. Drupon Rinpoche, in conversation with the author, 2011.

Chapter 9: Embracing the Obstacles

1. Antti Revonsuo, *Horizon: Why Do We Dream?*, BBC TV, 21 February 2009

2. Ibid.

3. Cited ibid.

4. Dr Pasang Yongten Arya, www.tibetanmedicine-edu.org/pdf/dreamsD1.pdf

5. Glenn H. Mullin, *Six Yogas of Naropa: Tsongkhapa's Commentary entitled: A Book of Three Inspirations*, Snow Lion Publications, 2005

6. Silvio Scarone, from the Università degli Studi di Milno, speaking at a European Science Foundation meeting in 2009, www.esf.org/activities/exploratory-workshops/news/ext-news-singleview/article/new-links-between-dreams-and-psychosis-could-revive-dream-therapy-in-psychiatry-585.html

7. J. Allan Hobson, *Dreaming*, Oxford University Press, 2005.

8. Hayashi, M., Hori, T., Masuda, A., 'The alerting effects of caffeine, bright light and face washing after a short daytime nap', *Clinical Neurophysiology*, 113 (2003), 2,268–78

9. www.ninds.nih.gov/disorders/brain_basics/understanding_sleep.htm

10. www.ncbi.nlm.nih.gov/pubmed/16782142

11. http://www.ninds.nih.gov/disorders/brain_basics/understanding_sleep.htm

12. http://news.bbc.co.uk/1/hi/magazine/8112619.stm

13. www.dailymail.co.uk/sciencetech/article-1375441/Dont-want-lie-Youre-probably-slim-optimistic-energetic--member-sleepless-elite.html

14. Hobson, op. cit.

15. www.sleepeducation.com/Disorder.aspx?id=16

16. http://news.bbc.co.uk/1/hi/wales/8364393.stm

17. Samuel Johnson, www.about-personal-growth.com/habit-quotes.html

18. John Greenleaf Whittier, 'Maud Muller', 1856

Chapter 10: Blurring the Boundaries

1. Glenn H. Mullin, *Six Yogas of Naropa: Tsongkhapa's Commentary entitled: A Book of Three Inspirations*, Snow Lion Publications, 2005.

2. Michael Katz, *Tibetan Dream Yoga*, Bodhi Tree, 2011, p.8

3. Ibid., p.40

4. C. G. Jung (ed.), *Man and his Symbols*, Aldus Books, 1964, p.37

5. http://www.guardian.co.uk/science/2011/feb/22/future-paranormality-richard-wiseman

6. Stowell, M. S., 'Precognitive dreams: a phenomenological study. Part I: Methodology and sample cases', *Journal of the American Society for Psychical Research,* 91 (1997), 163–220

7. Cited by Dr Larry Dossey, Scientific and Medical Network conference, Winchester University, April 2011

8. 'Precognitive Stock Market Dreamers', *Phenomena,* 1 November 2004

9. Dossey, op. cit.

10. Ibid.

11. Ibid.

12. http://www.dailymail.co.uk/sciencetech/article-452833/Is-REALLY-proof-man-future.html

13. http://science.nasa.gov/astrophysics/focus-areas/what-is-dark-energy/

14. http://www.dosseydossey.com/larry/links.html

15. Michael Katz, *Tibetan Dream Yoga*, Bodhi Tree, 2011, p.37

16. Dr Larry Dossey, Scientific and Medical Network conference, Winchester University, April 2011

17. Ibid.

18. Paul and Charla Devereux, *Lucid Dreaming*, Daily Grail Publishing, 2011, p.177

19. Arvid Guterstam, Arvid, Petkova, Valeria I., Ehrsonn, H. Henrik, 'The illusion of owning a third arm', PLoS ONE 6(2): e17208, online February 2011

20. Olivé, I., Berthoz, A., 'Combined Induction of Rubber-Hand Illusion and Out-of-Body Experiences', Laboratoire de Physiologie de la Perception et de l'Action, UMR 7152, College de France CNRS, Paris, France
21. Devereux, op. cit., p.175
22. http://www.lucidity.com/NL32.OBEandLD.html
23. Ibid.
24. Published in his book *Flight of Mind*, Scarecrow Press, 1986
25. Thomas Campbell, *My Big TOE*, Lightning Strike Books, 2007, p.85.
26. Todd Acamesis, OBE workshop, March 2010
27. In conversation with the author, 2010.
28. Talking at the Scientific and Medical Network conference, Winchester University 2011.

Chapter 11: Beyond Lucidity

1. Timothy Freke teaching on gnosis, December, 2011
2. Fritjof Capra, *The Tao of Physics*, http://www.goodreads.com/quotes/75791-quantum-theory-thus-reveals-a-basic-oneness-of-the-universe
3. Christopher Potter, *You Are Here*, Windmill Press, 2010, p.51
4. Werner Heisenberg, *Physics and Philosophy*, Harper and Row, 1962, p.145
5. Quoted in Werner Heisenberg, *Physics and Beyond: Encounters and Conversations*, Allen and Unwin, 1971, p.206
6. Adyashanti teachings
7. Rob Nairn, *Tranquil Mind*, Kairon Press, 1994.
8. Pema Chödron, www.tricycle.com/feature/no-right-no-wrong
9. Nairn, op. cit.
10. Richard Wiseman, *59 Seconds*, Pan, 2010, p.199
11. www.ted.com/talks/ben_goldacre_battling_bad_science.html
12. Wiseman, op. cit., p.198
13. Dr Beau Lotto, *Horizon: Is Seeing Believing?*, BBC2, 8 January 2011
14. Dr. Gustav Kuhn, ibid.
15. Dr Beau Lotto, ibid.

16. Traleg Kyabgon Rinpoche, *Dream Yoga*, five-disc DVD set, E-Vam Buddhist Institute, 2008

17. Lama Yeshe Rinpoche, in conversation with the author, September 2012.

18. www.bbc.co.uk/news/health-11741350

19. http://www.scientificamerican.com/podcast/episode. cm?id=mediation-correlated-with-structure-11-02-22

20. Stephen Batchelor, *Buddhism Without Beliefs*, Riverhead Books, 1997, p.32

21. Dilgo Khyentse Rinpoche, www.tricycle.com/insights/city-dreams

22. Tenzin Rinpoche, London talk, November 2012

Chapter 12: Awakening within the Dream

1. Lama Yeshe Rinpoche in conversation with the author, June 2011

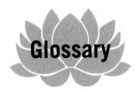

Glossary

the 4, 7, 8 Breath: a technique of regulating the breath in order to aid restful sleep.

the 4 a.m. demons: a psychological state characterized by anxiety or insecurity, which sometimes occurs upon awakening from sleep in the early hours.

bodhicitta: the mind of enlightenment, the wish to attain enlightenment for the benefit of all beings.

bodhisattva: a Sanskrit term for someone who has generated bodhicitta and whose life is devoted to helping all living beings to be free from suffering.

bodhisattva action: action encompassed by the six perfections of generosity, moral conduct, patience, joyful effort, meditation and wisdom.

Body and Breath technique: a variation of the FAC technique (*see below*) for entering the dream state lucidly.

circadian rhythms: physiological processes that occur in the course of a 24-hour period.

clear light experiences: experiences in which we encounter the true nature of our own mind, beyond our deluded projections of subject–object duality.

the clear light of sleep: a state of mind beyond all aspects of subject–object dualism, which occurs if we become super-lucid within the dreamless delta-wave stage of sleep.

the Columbo Method: a mindfulness-based awareness practice that can be engaged in both the waking and dream states in which we search for clues to our present state of consciousness and look closely at the surroundings, like the TV detective Lieutenant Columbo.

compensation: a Jungian term for inherent self-regulation in the psychic apparatus of the unconscious, which aims for harmonious balance within the psyche of both the accepted aspects of ourselves and the rejected aspects.

dream interpretation: assigning meaning to dreams through the process of decoding them for comprehension by the rational mind.

dream sign: any improbable, impossible or bizarre aspect of dream experience that can indicate that we are dreaming.

dream yoga: the union of consciousness within the dream and sleep states. Uses a series of practices, including advanced lucid dreaming methods, conscious sleeping techniques and what in the West is referred to as astral projection or OBE work on the path to spiritual awakening.

dreams of clarity: Tibetan Buddhist term for the class of dreams that include lucid dreams, witnessing dreams, dreams that contain significant insight and prophetic dreams.

FAC (Falling Asleep Consciously): a technique to enter either dreamless NREM2 or REM dreaming sleep without blacking out or losing conscious awareness.

false awakening: dreaming that we have woken up when we are in fact still dreaming.

fully lucid: the state of fully conscious reflective awareness within the dream, coupled with volitional interaction with the dreamscape and dream characters.

Hypnagogic Affirmation technique: requires that we pass through the hypnagogic state while mentally reciting a positive affirmation of our intent to gain lucidity.

Hypnagogic Drop-in technique: a variation of the FAC technique (*see above*) for entering the dream state lucidly.

hypnagogic hallucinations: similar to hypnagogic imagery (*see below*), but unique in that they are in rare cases superimposed onto our waking state experience.

hypnagogic imagery: mental images that flash and fade before our mind's eye as we drift off to sleep.

Hypnagogic Mindfulness technique (the 'Tao of Dozing'): a technique in which we maintain mindful awareness into the drowsy boundary of sleep.

hypnagogic state: the transitional state between wakefulness and sleep.

hypnopompic insights: flashes of inspiration and insight that occur in the hypnopompic state.

Hypnopompic Mindfulness technique ('Snooze Button Meditation'): a technique in which we maintain mindful awareness throughout the hypnopompic state.

hypnopompic state: the transitional state between sleep and full wakefulness.

joyful effort: enthusiastic effort for *dharma* practice; one of the Buddhist six perfections, the others being generosity, ethics, patience, concentration and wisdom.

lama: a Tibetan honorific title conferred on a Buddhist monk, nun or teacher.

life signs: triggers in waking life that can help us become more lucidly aware.

lucid dream: a dream in which we are actively aware that we are dreaming.

lucid dreaming: a form of mind training in which we learn to recognize our dreams as dreams while we are dreaming.

lucidity spectrum: spectrum based on the degrees of awareness within the dream, ranging from a suspicion that we might be dreaming to fully conscious reflective awareness.

Multiple Wake-ups technique: a technique where, after several hours of restful sleep, we are woken several times a night, hence have several chances to engage the lucid dreaming practices.

MILD (Mnemonic Initiated Lucid Dream): a lucid dreaming technique that works by using the functions of memory, self-hypnosis and visualization.

mindfulness: a meditation practice that could be defined as 'knowing what is happening while it is happening, without judgement or preference'.

Mindfulness of Dream & Sleep: a holistic approach to lucid dreaming and conscious sleeping which uses all areas of falling asleep, dreaming and waking up for spiritual and psychological growth.

myoclonic jerks: sudden spasms experienced as we enter NREM1 sleep.

nap: any short period of sleep outside the main sleep cycle.

NREM (non-rapid eye movement): NREM sleep is when we are not dreaming.

NREM1 (stage 1 non-REM sleep): experienced as drowsiness and often accompanied by alpha brainwave patterns of relaxed wakefulness, hypnagogic imagery and possibly myoclonic jerks.

NREM2 (stage 2 non-REM sleep): light, dreamless sleep that occurs once we experience the dissolution of external conscious awareness.

NREM3 (stage 3 non-REM sleep): the deepest level of usually dreamless sleep, during which our brain produces delta waves and we release human growth hormone, repair our cells and 'recharge the batteries'.

parasomnia: a category of sleep disorders that involve abnormal movements or behaviours.

pre-lucid: the state in which we critically question the reality of a dream.

pre-lucid confabulation: the process of talking ourselves out of becoming lucid while in the pre-lucid state.

the RAIN technique (Recognize, Allow, Intimate attention, Non-identification): a mindfulness meditation technique taught by the Mindfulness Association.

rainbow body: a level of spiritual realization often accompanied by the 'rainbow body phenomenon' in which the gross corporeal form of the physical body dissolves into coloured elemental light at the point of death, leaving nothing but the hair and fingernails behind.

REM: rapid eye movement during sleep, usually indicating dreaming.

REM debt: the phenomenon in which a lack of REM sleep is 'indebted' and then paid back during our next sleep cycle.

REM rebound: the process in which we experience elongated REM sleep periods if we have gone without REM sleep in our previous sleep cycle, or missed a sleep cycle entirely.

REM sleep behaviour disorder (RBD): a disorder whereby subjects physically act out their dreams as they are dreaming them.

rinpoche: an honorific Tibetan term meaning 'precious one'; usually reserved for high Lamas (see above) or masters.

samsara: a Buddhist term used to denote cyclic existence – the experience of birth, life, death and rebirth as perpetuated by ignorance.

samsaric dreams: dreams that reflect *samsara* (see *above*), consisting of habits, memories and desires from this life, and perhaps previous lives, too.

sankalpa: a statement of intent and a Sanskrit word meaning 'will, purpose or determination'.

semi-lucid: the state during which we experience lucid awareness but then slip back and forth between lucidity and non-lucidity.

the shadow: a Jungian concept used to describe the aspects of our psyche that we have unconsciously rejected, denied or disowned.

shadow integration: the practice of accepting and integrating the shadow.

shunyata: 'emptiness', a Buddhist term used to describe the impermanent and interdependent nature of all phenomena.

sleep paralysis: muscular paralysis caused by one of the three REM sleep states staying engaged while the other two (sensory blockade and cortical activation) have been disengaged, meaning that while our brain has partially woken up and our senses are taking in partial sensory input, our physical body cannot move.

sleepwalking: a parasomnia (see *above*) in which the subject engages in activities normally associated with wakefulness while in a sleep or sleep-like state.

somniloquy: sleeptalking, which is a type of parasomnia (see above), in which the subject makes coherent noises or speaks while in the sleep or dream states.

super-lucid: the highest level of awareness in the dream state; often characterized by an experience of partial non-dual awareness.

the unconscious: the totality of mind that lies beyond or beneath conscious awareness.

WILD (Wake Initiated Lucid Dream) technique: a well-known technique for entering the lucid dream state from the waking state without blacking out.

Weird technique: asking, 'Am I dreaming?' and checking into our present state of awareness whenever anything weird happens.

witnessing dream: a dream experienced lucidly from a gentle non-preferential perspective without any desire to influence or interact with it.

yidams: psychic archetypes of enlightened energy in the Tibetan Buddhist tradition, literally meaning 'mind-connection'.

yoga: union; see *also* dream yoga.

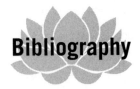

Bibliography

Valerie Austin, *Self-Hypnosis: A Step-by-Step Guide to Improving your Life*, Thorsons, 1994

Marc Barasch, *Healing Dreams*, Riverhead, 2000

Deirdre Barrett, *The Committee of Sleep*, Crown, 2001

Stephen Batchelor, *Buddhism without Beliefs: A Contemporary Guide to Awakening*, Riverhead Books, 1997

——, 'Buddhism for this one and only life', the first talk of his *Tricycle* online retreat, 26 June 2010

Fraser Boa, *The Way of the Dream: Conversations on Jungian Dream Interpretation with Marie Louise von Franz*, Windrose, 1988

Joseph Campbell, *The Inner Reaches of Outer Space*, A. van der Marck, 1986

Thomas Campbell, *My Big TOE: Awakenings, Discovery, Inner Workings: A Trilogy Unifying Philosophy, Physics, and Metaphysics*, Lightning Strike Books, 2007

Fritjof Capra, *The Tao of Physics: An Exploration of the Parallels Between Modern Physics and Eastern Mysticism*, Shambhala Publications, 1975

Carlos Castaneda, *Journey to Ixtlan: The Lessons of Don Juan*, Simon and Schuster, 1972

——, *The Art of Dreaming*, HarperCollins, 1994

Deepak Chopra, Debbie Ford presents *The Shadow Effect*, Hay House DVD, 2009

Lama Surya Das, *Tibetan Dream Yoga*, audio CD, Sounds True, 2001

Paul and Charla Devereux, *Lucid Dreaming: Accessing Your Inner Virtual Realities*, Daily Grail Publishing, 2011

Timothy Freke and Peter Gandy, *The Laughing Jesus*, Three Rivers Press, 2006

Sigmund Freud, *The Interpretation of Dreams*, trans. A. A. Brill, Macmillan, 1913; first published Franz Deuticke, 1899

Keith Hearne, *The Dream Machine*, The Aquarian Press, 1990

Werner Heisenberg, *Physics and Philosophy*, Harper and Row, 1962

—, *Physics and Beyond: Encounters and Conversations*, Allen and Unwin, 1971

J. Allan Hobson, *Dreaming: A Very Short Introduction*, Oxford University Press, 2005

Jim Horne, *Sleepfaring: A Journey through the Science of Sleep*, Oxford University Press 2006

H. J. Irwin, *Flight of Mind: A Psychological Study of the Out-of-Body Experience*, Scarecrow Press, 1986

C. G. Jung, 'The Importance of the Unconscious in Psychopathology', *The British Medical Journal*, vol. 2, no. 2,814 (5 December 1914), 964–8

—, *Archetypes and the Collective Unconscious*, Collected Works, Vol. 9, Part 1, Routledge and Kegan Paul, 1959

—, *Dreams*, trans. R. F. C. Hull, Princeton University Press, 1974

—, 'Psychology and Religion', 1938, in *Psychology and Religion: West and East*, Collected Works, Vol. 11, Princeton University Press, 1975

— (ed.), *Man and his Symbols*, Aldus Books, 1964

Michael Katz, *Tibetan Dream Yoga: The Royal Road to Enlightenment*, Bodhi Tree, 2011

Stephen LaBerge, PhD, *Lucid Dreaming*, Jeremy P. Tarcher, Inc., 1985

—, *Lucid Dreaming: A Concise Guide to Awakening in Your Dreams and in Your Life*, Sounds True, 2004

— and Howard Rheingold, *Exploring the World of Lucid Dreaming*, Ballantine Books, 1990

Daniel Love, *Are You Dreaming? Exploring Lucid Dreams: A Comprehensive Guide*, Enchanted Loom Publishing, 2013

Robert A. Monroe, *Journeys Out of the Body*, Doubleday, 1971

Glenn H. Mullin, *Six Yogas of Naropa: Tsongkhapa's Commentary entitled: A Book of Three Inspirations*, Snow Lion Publications, 2005

Rubin Naiman, PhD, *The Yoga of Sleep: Sacred and Scientific Practices to Heal Sleeplessness*, Sounds True, 2010

Rob Nairn, *Living, Dreaming, Dying: Practical Wisdom from the Tibetan Book of the Dead*, Shambhala Publications, 2004

—, *Tranquil Mind: An Introduction to Buddhism and Meditation*, Kairon Press, 1994

David N. Neubauer, *Understanding Sleeplessness*, The Johns Hopkins University Press, 2003

Chogyal Namkhai Norbu, *The Cycle of Day and Night: An Essential Tibetan Text on the Practice of Dzogchen*, Barrytown/Stationhill Press, 1987

—, *Dream Yoga and the Practice of Natural Light*, Snow Lion Publications, 2002

Christopher Potter, *You Are Here: A Portable History of the Universe*, Windmill Press, 2010

Rob Preece, *The Psychology of Buddhist Tantra*, Snow Lion Publications, 2012

David Richo, *Shadow Dance: Liberating the Power and Creativity of Your Dark Side*, Shambhala Publications, 1999

Dzigar Kongtrul Rinpoche, *It's Up to You*, Shambhala Publications, 2006

Dzogchen Ponlop Rinpoche, *Mind Beyond Death*, Snow Lion Publications, 2008

Gyaltrul Rinpoche, *Ancient Wisdom: Nyingma Teachings of Dream Yoga, Meditation and Transformation*, Snow Lion Publications, 1993

Namgyal Rinpoche, *The Womb of Form: Pith Instructions in the Six Yogas of Naropa*, Bodhi Publishing, 1998

Patrul Rinpoche, *Words of My Perfect Teacher: A Complete Translation of a Classic Introduction to Tibetan Buddhism*, trans. The Padmakara Translation Group, Shambhala Publications, 1994

Tenzin Wangyal Rinpoche, *The Tibetan Yogas of Dream and Sleep*, Snow Lion Publications, 1998

Traleg Kyabgon Rinpoche, *Dream Yoga*, five-disc DVD set, E-Vam Buddhist Institute, 2008.

G. Scott Sparrow, *Lucid Dreaming: Dawning of the Clear Light*, ARE Press, 1976

Jill Bolte Taylor, *My Stroke of Insight: A Brain Scientist's Personal Journey*, Hodder and Stoughton, 2008

Frederick van Eeden, 'A study of dreams', *Proceedings of the Society for Psychical Research*, 1913

Francisco J. Varela and HH Dalai Lama, *Sleeping, Dreaming, and Dying: An Exploration of Consciousness with the Dalai Lama*, Wisdom Publications, 1997

Robert Waggoner, *Lucid Dreaming: Gateway to the Inner Self*, Moment Point Press, 2009

B. Alan Wallace, *Dreaming Yourself Awake: Lucid Dreaming and Tibetan Dream Yoga for Insight and Transformation*, Shambhala Publications, 2012

Jeff Warren, *Head Trip: A Fantastic Romp through 24 Hours in the Life of your Brain*, Oneworld Publications, 2009

Richard Wiseman, *59 Seconds: Think a Little, Change a Lot*, Pan, 2010

W. B. Yeats, *Responsibilities*, Cuala Press, 1914

Serenity Young, *Dreaming in the Lotus: Buddhist Narrative, Imagery and Practice*, Wisdom Publications, 1999

Acknowledgements

I would like to express my gratitude to all the people who have helped me write this book and helped me be everything I can be.

But first of all I would like to contextualize the process a little bit. This book was written on planes, trains and Buddhist centre floors over the course of three years as I gradually faded out of the music and dance scene and into full-time lucidity teaching. It was my mentor, Rob Nairn, who suggested that I write a book and who was in fact the editor of the first draft back in 2010. Once Rob was convinced that I wasn't saying anything too outlandish, he guided me into the capable hands of Erika van Greunen and the amazing Albert Buhr, who spent months cutting, polishing and refining the text. (Albert wears Wellington boots to nightclubs so that he's 'prepared for anything'. Now that's what you want in an editor!) Once Albert had done all he could, the manuscript landed up at Hay House with the wonderful Lizzie Hutchins, who continued the editing process.

Although there have been many people who have helped me with this book, I take full responsibility for any errors or inaccuracies within the text and I apologize for any and all of these.

Acknowledgements

There are so many people who deserve thanks and gratitude in regard to making this book happen that I am sure to have forgotten a few, but among those I can remember I offer my heartfelt thanks to:

Mantis Clan and my friends from Kingston for helping me grow up so happily.

The THROWDOWN team and every one of the dancers and dance lovers who supported us over the amazing decade I spent in the hip-hop scene.

Donna Dee for showing me the way.

Greg for the front cover artwork and everything you do.

Stuart Mullins and Theatre is, Emma and Davyd from Gateways of the Mind, Lisa for the theatre tours, Phil Evans for the pilgrimage, Terry Nicholls for seeing past my ego, Rob Davis for being my first sensei, and Choden for saying the fateful words 'Your lucid dream practice sounds interesting. You should go and talk to Rob Nairn about it.'

Rob Castell for the writing retreats in Cadaques and for the constant support.

Debbie Winterbourne, Sally Muir, John Lockley, Todd Acamesis, Rory MacSweeney, Caroline McCready, Robert Waggoner, Sergio Mangaña and all the other dream teachers I have had the privilege of working with.

Danni and the One Taste team.

Rob Nairn and all the Mindfulness Association teachers.

The London lucid dreaming scene for their bedrock of support.

The late Mervyn Minall-Jones for teaching me self-hypnosis.

Erika for all the hard work in the early stages of the project and for the opportunity you gave me.

Ya'Acov Darling Khan and Tim Freke for opening the door to Hay House, and Michelle Pilley for letting me in.

Stephen LaBerge, Keith Hearne and all the other daring outliers.

All those who kindly read through sections of the final draft and offered corrections and advice, including the lovely Robert Waggoner, Graham Nicholls, Josep Soler, Dr Alan Taylor, Fay Adams and of course Albert Buhr once more.

Special thanks go to Georgina Hamilton, without whom this book would simply not have happened, and to all the sangha of South Africa and Zimbabwe for their ongoing support.

Thanks to Koelle Simpson and the rest of Martha Beck's 'life coach dreamers' and to Lisa Tran for the opportunity at TED.

Huge thanks to my mum, dad, brother and family members (old and new), who have been so supportive throughout.

Thank you to my fiancée, Jade, and to the family that we will one day have.

To Lama Zangmo and all the London Samye Dzong sangha, and to all the Samye Dzong centres at which I have had the privilege to teach.

To my dreams and to the hypnopompic state in which I composed many of the key points of this book.

To my teachers Lama Yeshe Rinpoche, Akong Rinpoche, Rob Nairn and Lama Zangmo for their kindness and patience with me.

To Rigpa and Sogyal Rinpoche for those first vital steps along the path.

To Amy, Michelle, Jo, Ruth, Jessica, Julie and the rest of the brilliant team at Hay House for all their hard work.

And finally, thank *you* for taking the time to read this book. I sincerely hope that it benefits you in some way and that it encourages you to follow your dreams, as I did through writing it.

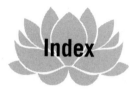

Index

ABOUT THE AUTHOR

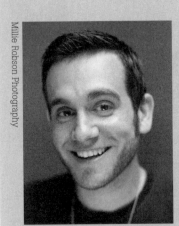

Charlie Morley has been a self-taught lucid dreamer since the age of 17 and a practising Buddhist for the past 10 years, after taking refuge with Akong Rinpoche. In 2008, at the age of 25, Charlie started teaching lucid dreaming within the context of Tibetan Buddhism at the request of his mentor, the well-known meditation instructor Rob Nairn.

Soon after he started teaching, Charlie received the traditional Tibetan Buddhist 'authorization to teach' from his guru, Lama Yeshe Rinpoche, which was not only a great honour but also a valuable seal of approval from such a highly regarded lama.

In 2010 Charlie and Rob Nairn began to pioneer a new holistic approach to lucid dreaming and conscious sleeping called Mindfulness of Dream & Sleep. Since then Charlie has run lucid dreaming workshops and Mindfulness of Dream & Sleep retreats around the UK, Europe, Africa and America. He has featured on BBC Radio 4 and lectured at Goldsmiths University, London, Cape Town Medical School and the Royal Geographical Society. In 2011 he gave the first ever TED talk on lucid dreaming at a conference in San Diego.

Before being asked to teach lucid dreaming, Charlie had completed a BA honours degree in drama, which led him to work as an actor, a scriptwriter and even a rapper in a Buddhist hip-hop group. Alongside this, he was the manager and company director of Throwdown, a collective of breakdancers and hip-hop artists who toured extensively round Europe.

Charlie currently lives at Kagyu Samye Dzong Buddhist Centre in London with his fiancée, Jade. He has a 1st Dan blackbelt in kickboxing and enjoys parkour, surfing and dreaming!

www.charliemorley.com